Menu Me!

28 Day Diabetes Meal Planner-

Lower Carb Menus & Easy Recipes

Text Copyright © 2016

All Rights Reserved

Easyhealth LLC

PREFACE

This book of calorie and carb controlled menus is written with the purpose of helping those who have been placed on a modified carbohydrate diet by their health professional and are looking for meal planning ideas. The ideal situation would be to ask your health provider for a referral to a Registered Dietitian to assist you with individualized meal plan development. The generalized menus provided in this book are a springboard to help you as you learn to adjust to your healthcare professional's recommended diet plan. If you do not know your daily carbohydrate and or calorie goals, contact your healthcare team for advice. It is very important to communicate with your healthcare provider and your diabetes care team to properly care for any individual with diabetes. If your healthcare provider has placed you on a specific calorie level (such as 1500 calories, 1800 calories, etc.), you may find one of the many other Easyhealth Nutrition ebooks helpful also. You may find our other titles on our Amazon author page- just search Easyhealth Nutrition.

This book is not intended to diagnose or treat any medical condition or as a substitute for the medical advice of a physician. Readers should consult with their health professional with regard to matters of health and/or symptoms which would require a physician's advice. Always consult with your physician before making any changes in your diet, exercise or health routines.

TABLE OF CONTENTS

28 Day Diabetes Meal Planner- 1

Lower Carb Menus & Easy Recipes 1

PREFACE 3

TABLE OF CONTENTS 4

MEAL PLANNING 101 7

PORTION CONTROL 9

ASK THE DIETITIAN 10

CARB CONTROLLED MENUS 12

    APPROX 30GM CARB/MEAL 13
        WEEK 1 13
        WEEK 2 16
        WEEK 3 18
        WEEK 4 20

    APPROX 45GM CARB/MEAL 24
        WEEK 1 24
        WEEK 2 27
        WEEK 3 29
        WEEK 4 32

    APPROX 60GM CARB/MEAL 36
        WEEK 1 36
        WEEK 2 39
        WEEK 3 42
        WEEK 4 45

EASY RECIPES 49

    SALADS 49
        CAESAR SALAD 49
        CARIBBEAN COLESLAW 49
        COBB SALAD PLATTER 50
        COLESLAW 50
        EASY GREEK CHICKEN SALAD BOWL 50
        GREEK CHICKEN CHOPPED SALAD 51
        SPINACH SALAD 51
        SUMMER CORN SALAD 52
        TACO SALAD 52

    SANDWICHES AND WRAPS 53
        APPLE NUT SANDWICH 53

CHEESE TOAST	53
GREEK CHICKEN SALAD STUFFED PITA	53
GREEK CHICKEN SANDWICH	54
GREEK CHICKEN WRAP	54
GRILLED SHRIMP WRAP	55
TURKEY SWISS WRAP	55
EGGS AND BREAKFAST DISHES	**56**
BREAKFAST BANANA SPLIT	56
BREAKFAST BURRITO	56
CHEESY EGGS	57
CINNAMON TOAST	57
COUNTRY EGG SANDWICH	57
DEVILED EGGS	58
EASY EGGS	58
EGG BAKED IN AVOCADO CUPS	59
EGGS BENEDICT	59
EGGS IN HAM CUPS	59
ENGLISH MUFFIN STACK	60
FRENCH TOAST	60
GREEK YOGURT PARFAIT	61
HAM, EGG AND VEGGIE ROLL UP	61
HIGH PROTEIN OATMEAL	62
OAT BOWL	62
OATMEAL BANANA SMOOTHIE	62
SWEET POTATO BREAKFAST CUPS	63
VEGGIE OMELET	63
MAIN DISHES	**65**
BALSAMIC PORK TENDERLOIN	65
CHICKEN (OR PORK) & VEGGIE STIR FRY	65
CRUNCHY FISH TACOS WITH CARIBBEAN SLAW	66
EASY BAKED FISH	66
EASY GREEK CHICKEN	67
EGGPLANT PARM	67
FAVORITE TACOS	68
FLATBREAD PIZZA	68
FRIED RICE	69
GREEK CHICKEN SALAD	69
GRILLED BBQ PORK CHOP	69
HERB ROASTED CHICKEN & VEGGIES	70
HUMMUS LUNCH BOWL	70
JERK CHICKEN	71
LIGHTER LASAGNA CAPRESE	71

OPEN FACED LOADED BURGERS 72
OVEN BAKED BBQ RIBS 72
PATTY MELT WITH CARAMELIZED ONIONS 72
PINEAPPLE GRILLED CHICKEN 73
PORK & SPANISH RICE 73
PORK TENDERLOIN WITH APPLES 74
RED & WHITE CHICKEN CHILI 75
ROTISSERIE CHICKEN 75
SALMON PATTIES 76
STEAK KABOBS 76
TORTILLA PIZZA 77
TURKEY DIVAN 77
TURKEY MEATSAUCE 78
VERACRUZ STYLE SNAPPER 78

VEGETABLES AND SIDE DISHES **80**
BALSAMIC MUSHROOMS 80
BROCCOLI TOSS 80
POTATO SKINS 80
RAW VEGGIE PLATE 81
ROASTED CHERRY TOMATOES 81
ROASTED GREEN BEANS WITH ONIONS 82
ROASTED VEGGIES 82

DESSERTS **83**
BAKED APPLES 83
BAKED PEARS 83
BANANA ICE CREAM 84
BERRIES WITH COCONUT AND WHIPPED CREAM 84
BLUEBERRY CRISP 84
CHOCOLATE BERRIES 85

MISCELLANEOUS **86**
BBQ RUB SEASONING 86
BERRY CRUSH 86
EASY MARINARA SAUCE 86
PARMESAN CRISPS 87
SMALL BATCH CORNBREAD 87

RECIPE INDEX **88**

MEAL PLANNING 101

What should a Type 2 diabetes diet consist of?

The type 2 diabetes diet should contain proper amounts of carbohydrate, protein and fats. Carbohydrate foods include corn, peas, bread, fruit and milk. Protein foods include meat, poultry, fish, eggs and cheese. Examples of fats are mayonnaise, butter, sour cream, salad dressing and nuts. A properly planned diet also includes variety to provide proper vitamins and minerals. In other words, the "diabetic diet" is a safe, healthy way of eating for you and your family.

Where do I start?

Hopefully, your doctor or healthcare provider gave you a carbohydrate level to follow or a carbohydrate range to stay within. If not, ask for their advice regarding your specific carbohydrate/calorie needs based on your height, weight, age, activity level and glucose goals. A goal of Type 2 diabetes control may be weight loss, if needed, and exercise. Weight loss and exercise will help your body metabolize your food more efficiently. **Ask your healthcare provider for approval before you change your diet and/or exercise habits.**

Should I count calories or carbs?

It depends. If you need to lose weight, count calories and carbs. If you are already at a proper weight, count carbs. Carb counting diets may be higher in calories, especially if you are not watching your protein and/or fat intake. Be sure to monitor your weight and adjust your calorie intake as needed for weight maintenance. The menus included in this ebook show you both calories and carb amounts since many people with type 2 diabetes benefit from even a modest weight loss. Feel free to mix and match the breakfast, lunch and supper menus that best meet your specific needs as recommended by your healthcare provider.

Should I eliminate carbs completely?

While it is important to monitor carb intake, do not completely eliminate them from your diet. Many healthful foods contain carbs such as beans, peas, whole grains, fruit and low fat dairy. The key is portion control. Remember, though, each person may respond slightly differently to any particular carbohydrate food. You will want to monitor your glucose frequently to help you learn which carbs work best for you. Generally, most people will do best when they choose and measure carbs with extra fiber such as fruit, beans, peas, whole grains, and vegetables etc. rather than juice, processed foods and high sugar foods.

What about protein and fat?

Protein and fat do not contain carbohydrate, so they generally do not increase glucose levels. Choose protein sources like skinless chicken, fish, lean beef, eggs, and cheese. Fat choices include nuts, seeds, mayonnaise, oils, avocado and olives. Baking, broiling, boiling or grilling your food will help keep calories lower than frying or sautéing foods.

PORTION CONTROL

Getting a handle on proper carb portion sizes is essential to lowering glucose and/or losing weight. Learning portions at home will help you estimate your portion sizes more accurately when you are eating out. Each menu shows carb amounts for the portion listed. Please note that carbs may vary between brands and manufacturers, so be sure to check labels and adjust your portion size accordingly. Let's look at general information regarding portion sizes:

Carbohydrates: You will generally choose 2-4 serving of carb per meal depending on your health professional's carb level recommendation.

> Starchy vegetables- generally a serving is 1/3 -1/2 cup of cooked pasta, rice, beans, corn.
> Non-Starchy Vegetables- generally a "free food" due to low carb content.
> Fruit- one small fruit, ½ cup canned fruit or 1/3 to 1/2 cup juice is one serving
> Milk- 1 cup milk or 6 oz. yogurt is one serving
> Other carbs- foods which contain carbs but do not fit previous categories such as sugar free ice cream, sugar free pudding, sauces, light jelly, etc. (see "other carbohydrates" heading for serving sizes)

Protein: You will generally choose 1 or more servings of protein at each meal depending upon your goals for your weight.

> Meat, fish, poultry- a rough estimate of portion size is equal to the palm of your hand.
> Cheese- generally 1-2 oz.
> Eggs- Egg yolks contain many vitamins and minerals for health. Egg whites are an excellent source of lean protein.
> Peanut Butter- 1 Tbsp.

Fat: You will generally choose at least one serving of fat at each meal, depending upon your goals for your weight.

> Oils, margarine, butter, mayonnaise- 1 tsp.- 1 Tbsp.
> Salad Dressings- 1-3 Tbsp.
> Nuts- small handful
> Olives- 8-10
> Avocado, Sour Cream- 2 Tbsp.

ASK THE DIETITIAN

What can I drink with my meals? The best beverage is one that contains few carbs such as water, unsweetened tea, water with lemon juice, etc. Avoid sweetened beverages such as soda, sweet tea, lemonade, sports drinks and energy beverages. If you choose to drink juice, be sure to measure carefully as juice is very high in carbs. Check the food labels on non-dairy and dairy beverages and measure accordingly.

What will make my blood glucose go up besides too many carbs? Several factors can cause an increase in glucose levels. If you have an illness or infection, your glucose may rise. Also, stress can cause a rise in glucose levels. It is important to realize that you will not achieve diabetes management perfection each and every day. Don't stress about occasional glucose spikes. You should be more concerned if your glucose levels stay high on a weekly basis rather than the short lived high that occurs here and there. If you are doing all you can with your diet and you still have high glucose levels- see your doctor. You may need a medication adjustment to prevent damage to your body from constantly elevated glucose levels.

No more fast food? In general, fast food carbs are more processed, so they will tend to increase glucose levels more than a meal of high fiber carbs. Try to limit the times you go for fast food by learning how to make "copycat" versions of your favorite fast foods at home. You can tweak recipes by adding various seasonings, etc. to up the fiber and nutrition. When you do eat out, visit the restaurant's website first to find nutrition information regarding carbs, etc. This will help you make better choices and control portion sizes. You will probably need to bring home part of your meal for use later to avoid overeating. If you do splurge, take a walk when you get home to help lower your glucose levels. If you are having trouble controlling your intake when dining out, consider having a salad or a bowl of soup at home before leaving for the restaurant.

What are the best foods for diabetes? Foods which are high fiber, lower fat, vitamin rich and minimally processed make the best choices for a diabetes meal plan. Think brightly colored fruits and vegetables, lean protein, fish, beans, peas, low-fat yogurt and flaxseed just to name a few. All of these are included in the sample menus.

Are there any certain foods I must avoid? Many people with diabetes report difficulty controlling their glucose levels when they eat certain foods. Those foods are usually highly processed and/or contain excessive sugar. Examples of some of these foods to avoid are fast food French fries, cakes, pies, regular sodas, purchased smoothies, purchased burgers and fried meat sandwiches and sports beverages.

Can diabetes be cured? Unfortunately there is currently no cure for diabetes, although it CAN be controlled. The key components to control include diet, exercise and medication (if needed). Some people are able to control their glucose levels by losing weight and exercising. Even though their glucose levels are normal, they still have diabetes which would re-occur if the weight returned or if they quit exercising.

CARB CONTROLLED MENUS

The menus are set up to provide a consistent carb level at each meal, but feel free to pick and choose meals between the various carb levels if your health provider has you follow a different carb level at each meal. **Always consult with your healthcare provider before making any changes in your eating habits!**

As you work your way through the menus, you will note a variety of recipes including very simple ones for foods such as cheese toast, salads, etc. By having a recipe for these simple foods, it allows a better analysis of the carb level of the recipe. Hopefully, you will find ALL the recipes to be quite easy so that even those who possess little or no cooking skills will be able to prepare basic, delicious meals while controlling their carb intake.

Carbohydrate data is listed for each recipe and menu suggestion. Please note that non-starchy vegetables may be included in the diet as a "free food" (no carbs) up to 3 cups raw or 1 ½ cups cooked at a meal. Because of this, many of the salad and veggie recipes do not count toward your carb allotment for that meal. These foods contain a high amount of fiber which helps to control glucose levels. Try to include these foods often in your diet.

<u>Please note that underlined meal items are recipes found in this book.</u>

APPROX 30GM CARB/MEAL

WEEK 1

1. *Breakfast 293 calories/28.5gm carb/14gm pro*
   Easy Eggs- 1 Serving (.5gm carb)
   Fresh or Frozen (no sugar added) Strawberries- 1 ¼ cup whole berries (15gm carb)
   English Muffin, Whole Wheat- ½ muffin (13gm carb)
   Butter, Light -1 Tbsp.
   Lunch 638 calories/28.5 gm carb/45gm pro
   Easy Greek Chicken Salad Bowl- 1 serving
   Blueberries- ½ cup (11 gm carb)
   Ranch Salad Dressing 2 Tablespoons- (4.5gm carb)
   Diced Avocado- ¼ cup – (3 gm carb)
   Thin Wheat Crackers- 8 (10gm carb)
   Dinner 499 calories/28gm carb/36gm pro
   Grilled BBQ Pork Chop- 1 serving (1gm carb)
   Coleslaw- 3 oz. (8gm carb)
   Deviled Eggs - 2 halves (2gm carb)
   Whole Kernel Corn- ½ cup- (17gm carb)

2. *Breakfast 235 calories/30gm carb/13gm pro*
   Country Egg Sandwich – 1 serving (20 gm carb)
   Tangerines- 1 small (10 gm carb)
   Lunch 419 calories/28gm carb/21gm pro
   Flatbread Pizza (28 gm carb)
   Dinner 684 calories/29.5gm carb/61gm pro
   Steamed Shrimp- 8 oz. (1 gm carb)
   Tossed Salad -1 cup lettuce/ ½ cup cherry tomatoes
   Ranch Salad Dressing- 3 Tbsp. (2.5gm carb)
   Sunflower Seeds salad topping-1 Tbsp. (2gm carb)
   Thin Wheat Crackers-10- (14gm carb)
   Cantaloupe -3/4 cup cubes (10 gm carb)

3. *Breakfast 227 calories/32gm carb/12gm pro*
   Greek Yogurt Parfait -1 serving -(31 gm carb)
   Lunch 542 calories/28.5gm carb/45gm pro
   Greek Chicken Salad – 5.5 oz. (2gm carb) on
     2 Slices Thin Bread (16gm carb)
   Lettuce- 1/3 cup / Tomato- 1 slice
   Light Mayonnaise-1 Tbsp.- (1.5gm carb)
   Baby Carrots- 4 medium-
   Low Carb Yogurt- 12 oz. (9 gm carb)
   Dinner 758calories/32gm carb/43gm pro
   Grilled Sirloin Steak- 3 oz. with Balsamic Mushrooms
   Roasted Veggies
   Potato Skins- 1 serving (12gm carb)
   Berries with Coconut and Whipped Cream (20gm carb)

4. *Breakfast 195 calories/30.5gm carb/12gm pro*
   Oat Bowl- 1 serving (15gm carb)
   Canadian Bacon- 2 slices (.5gm carb)
   Raisins- 2 Tablespoons- (15gm carb)
   Lunch 603 calories/30gm carb/32gm pro
   Open-Faced Veggie & Beef Burger – 1 serving (14gm carb)
   Sweet Potato Chips-12 chips or 1 oz. (15gm carb)
   Dinner 506 calories/33gm carb/41gm pro
   Favorite Tacos- 2 tacos (33gm carb)

5. *Breakfast 294 calories/29.5gm carb/10gm pro*
   Easy Eggs- 1 serving (.5gm carb)
   Raisin Bread (unfrosted)-1 slice (14gm carb)
   Sliced Strawberries- ½ cup (6gm carb)
   Fruit Spread, 100% fruit-1 Tablespoon (9gm carb)
   Butter or Margarine- 1 Tablespoon
   Lunch 534 calories/30gm carb/30gm pro
   Meatballs- 4 medium (6gm carb)
   Whole wheat pasta- ½ cup (18.5gm carb)
   Easy Marinara Sauce- 4 oz. (5gm carb)
   Broccoli Toss – ½ cup
   Parmesan Cheese, grated -2 Tablespoons (.5gm carb)

Dinner 434 calories/29gm carb/22gm pro
Easy Baked Fish- 3oz.
Baked Sweet Potato-medium 5 oz. - (29gm carb)
Butter or Margarine- 1 Tablespoon
Spinach Salad - 2oz.

6. *Breakfast 356 calories/31gm carb/31gm pro*
   Pork Tenderloin, broiled- 3 oz.
   Oat Bowl- 1 serving (14.5gm carb)
   Raisins- 2 Tablespoons (14 gm carb)
   Flaxseed -ground- 1 Tbsp. -add to oat bowl (2.5gm carb)
   Lunch 601 calories/28gm carb/37gm pro
   Tomato Soup- 8 oz. (15gm carb)
   Cheese Toast -1 serving (8 gm carb)
   Tossed Salad w/turkey ham,cheese-1 ½ cups
   Salad Dressing- 2 Tablespoons (5 gm carb)
   Dinner 386 calories/28.5gm carb/43gm pro
   Turkey Divan- 1 serving (10gm carb)
   Brown Rice- 1/3 cup cooked (15gm carb)
   Dark Chocolate-6 gm (3.5gm carb)

7. *Breakfast 445 calories/29gm carb/30gm pro*
   Breakfast Burrito-1 serving (17gm carb)
   Grapes- ¾ cup (12gm carb)
   Lunch 332 calories/31gm carb/20gm pro
   Tuna Salad- ½ cup (9.5gm carb) with celery, baby carrots, tomato slices
   Thin Wheat Crackers-12 (16gm carb)
   Tomato, Fresh- 2 slices
   Cantaloupe- 1/8th of a medium melon (5.5 gm carb)
   Dinner 347 calories/29gm carb/43gm pro
   Herb-Roasted Chicken & Veggies – 1 serving
   Whole Kernel Corn- ½ cup (15gm carb)
   Canned Peaches, Juice Pack- ½ cup (14gm carb)

WEEK 2

8. *Breakfast 217 calories/29gm carb/11gm pro*
   Oatmeal Banana Smoothie (28gm carb)
   Almonds, roasted- 1 Tablespoons (1gm carb)
   Lunch 472 calories/30gm carb/46gm pro
   Greek Chicken Sandwich (22 gm carb)
   Vegetable Soup- 1 cup (8gm carb)
   Dinner 441 calories/30.5gm carb/33gm pro
   Balsamic Pork Tenderloin- 4.5gm serving (1.5gm carb)
   Small Baked Sweet Potato- 5 oz. (29gm Carb)
   Butter or Margarine- 1 Tablespoon
   Spinach Salad

9. *Breakfast 271 calories/29gm carb/10gm pro*
   English muffin- ½ (13.5gm carb)
   Butter or Margarine- 1 Tablespoon
   Poached Egg-1
   Blueberries- ¾ cup (15.5gm carb)
   Lunch 724 calories/29gm carb/50gm pro
   Steak Kabobs- 1 serving or 10 oz.
   Tossed Salad w/ham, turkey, cheese- 1 ½ cup
   Ranch Dressing- 2 Tablespoons (1.5gm carb)
   Wild Rice, cooked- ½ cup (18gm carb)
   Plums, sliced- ½ cup (9.5 gm carb)
   Dinner 264 calories/30gm carb/15gm pro
   Eggplant Parm- 1 serving (11.5gm carb)
   Whole Wheat Pasta- ½ cup (18.5gm carb)
   Olives, Black, chopped- 3 Tablespoons

10. *Breakfast 394 calories/31gm carb/21gm pro*
    French Toast – 1 serving (23gm carb)
    Berry Crush- 1 serving (8gm carb)
    Bacon- 2 slices
    Butter- 1 Tablespoon
    Lunch 552 calories/32gm carb/38gm pro
    Chef's Salad w/cheese, egg, turkey, ham, lettuce, tomato
    Grapes, 17 small (15gm carb)
    Whole Wheat Croutons- 2/3 cup (14 gm carb)
    Salad Dressing, Light-3 Tablespoons (3gm carb)

Dinner   306 calories/28gm carb/29gm pro
Roast Beef Sandwich on thin whole wheat bread (20 gm carb)
with lettuce & tomato
Honey mustard dressing- 2 Tablespoons (8gm carb)
Gazpacho Soup- 1 cup

11. *Breakfast   306 calories/29gm carb/17gm pro*
    Oat Bowl- 1 serving (15gm carb)
    Ham, Egg and Veggie Roll Up -1 serving
    Raisins-2 Tablespoons (14gm carb)
    Lunch   380 calories/28.5gm carb/32gm pro
    Greek Chicken Salad Stuffed Pita – 1 serving (13 gm carb)
    Honeydew Melon, cubed- 1 cup (15.5 gm carb)
    Dinner   511 calories/29gm carb/37gm pro
    Fried Rice – 1 serving (24.5gm carb)
    Cashews- ½ oz. or 8-10 (4.5gm carb)

12. *Breakfast   397 calories/29gm carb/24gm pro*
    Raisin bread, unfrosted- 1 slice (16 gm carb)
    Eggs in Ham Cups- 1 serving
    2% milk- 1 cup (12gm carb)
    Cream Cheese- 2 Tablespoons (1gm carb)
    Lunch 242 calories/28gm carb/17gm pro
    Crunchy Fish Tacos with Caribbean Slaw - 1 serving (28gm carb)
    Dinner 625 calories/29gm carb/27gm pro
    Chili with beans- ¾ cup (24gm carb)
    Sour Cream- 2 Tablespoons (2gm carb)
    Cheddar Cheese, shredded- 2 oz. (1gm carb)
    Side Salad- 3 oz.
    Ranch Dressing- 2 Tablespoons (2gm carb)

13. *Breakfast 297 calories/31gm carb/9 gm pro*
    Apple-Nut Sandwich (31 gm carb)
    Lunch 542 calories/29gm carb/40gm pro
    Turkey Swiss Wrap (25gm carb)
    Avocado Cubed, 1/3 cup (4gm carb)
    Dinner 475 calories/30gm carb/43gm pro
    Spinach Salad with Grilled Shrimp- 5 oz.
    Strawberries, sliced- 1 1/3 cup (16.5gm carb)
    Whipped Cream- 2 Tablespoons (1gm carb)
    Dark Chocolate Bar, miniature- 3 bars (12.5gm carb)

14. *Breakfast 292 calories/29.5gm carb/17gm pro*
Eggs Benedict - serving (17 gm carb)
Fresh Peach, small (12.5 gm carb)
Lunch 272 calories/31gm carb/14gm pro
Tortilla Pizza -1 serving (23.5gm carb)
Grapes, frozen- ½ cup (7.5gm carb)
Dinner 702 calories/32gm carb/44gm pro
Salmon Pattie- 2 servings (12gm carb)
Coleslaw - 1 serving (8gm carb)
Potato Skins- 1 serving (12gm carb)

WEEK 3

15. *Breakfast 282 calories/31gm carb/21gm pro*
Breakfast Banana Split- 1 serving (31gm carb)
Lunch 377 calories/31gm carb/25gm pro
Red & White Chicken Chili- 1 serving (30gm carb)
Sour Cream- 2 Tablespoons (1gm carb)
Cheddar Cheese, shredded- 1 oz.
Dinner 420 calories/31gm carb/39gm pro
Jerk Chicken
Caribbean Coleslaw- 1 serving
Roasted Sweet Potatoes- ½ cup (12.5gm carb)
Mango, diced- ¾ cup (18.5gm carb)
Butter or margarine- 1 Tablespoon

16. *Breakfast 296 calories/29.5gm carb/16gm pro*
Oat Bowl with Cinnamon- 1 serving (14.5 gm carb)
Small Apple- sliced (15gm carb)
Boiled Egg-2
Lunch 362 calories/29gm carb/34gm pro
Greek Chicken Wrap – 1 serving (13gm carb)
Blueberries- ¾ cup (16gm carb)
Dinner 336 calories/29gm carb/19gm pro
Lighter Lasagna Caprese- 1 serving (29gm carb)

17. *Breakfast 379 calories/29gm carb/32gm pro*
Pork Tenderloin, grilled – 3 oz.
Cinnamon Toast- 1 serving (20gm carb)
Small Banana- ½ (9 gm carb)

Lunch 688 calories/29.5gm carb/58gm pro
Cobb Salad Platter – 1 serving (3gm carb)
Ranch Salad Dressing -2 Tablespoons (5gm carb)
Crackers, Multigrain, 4 crackers (9.5gm carb)
Grapes- ¾ cup (12gm carb)
Dinner 336 calories/30.5gm carb/24gm pro
Pork Tenderloin with Apples -1 serving (10.5gm carb)
Green Beans- 1 cup
Sweet Potato, baked- 1 medium-3.5oz. (20gm carb)
Butter or Margarine- 1 Tablespoon

18. *Breakfast 400 calories/31gm carb/12gm pro*
Egg Baked in Avocado Cups – 1 serving (9gm carb)
Whole Wheat English Muffin- ½ (14gm carb)
Grapes- ½ cup (8gm carb)
Butter or Margarine- 1 Tablespoon
Lunch 606 calories/30.5gm carb/29gm pro
Beef & Vegetable Soup -10 oz. (14gm carb)
Cheese Toast- 2 serving (16gm carb)
Side Salad- 6 oz.
Bacon & Tomato Salad Dressing- 2 Tablespoons (.5gm carb)
Dinner 351 calories/30.5gm carb/28gm pro
Veracruz Style Snapper – 1 serving
Lima Beans- ¾ cup (30.5gm carb)

19. *Breakfast 265 calories/29gm carb/8gm pro*
High Protein Oatmeal - 1 serving (15gm carb)
Raisins- 2 Tablespoons (14gm carb)
Butter or Margarine- 1 Tablespoon
Lunch 319 calories/28gm carb/26gm pro
Grilled Shrimp Wrap – 1 serving (28gm carb)
Dinner 444 calories/30gm carb/40gm pro
Oven Baked BBQ Ribs -1 serving
Baked Beans, lower sugar- ½ cup (22gm carb)
Butter or Margarine- 1 Tablespoon
Coleslaw – 1 serving (8gm carb)

20. *Breakfast 386 calories/28.5gm carb/16gm pro*
    5 Grain Cooked Cereal or oatmeal- ½ cup (15gm carb)
    2 Tablespoons Raisins (14.5gm carb)
    Cheesy Eggs- 1 serving
    Bacon, Baked- 2 strips
    Butter- 1 Tablespoon
    Lunch 578 calories/27.5 gm carb/36gm pro
    Chicken and Veggie Stir Fry -1 serving
    Sweet & Sour Sauce- 1 Tablespoon (6.5gm carb)
    Brown Rice- 1/3 cup (15gm carb)
    Peanuts- 1 ounce (6gm carb)
    Dinner 297 calories/28gm carb/12gm pro
    Beef Stew- 1 cup (15gm carb)
    Small Batch Cornbread- 1 serving (13gm carb)

21. *Breakfast 334 calories/31.5gm carb/18gm pro*
    English Muffin Stack – 1 serving (26gm carb)
    Low Sugar Jelly- 2 teaspoons (5.5gm carb)
    Lunch 627 calories/29.5gm carb/33gm pro
    Tuna Salad Stuffed Tomato- 6oz. (16gm carb)
    Thin Wheat Crackers-8 (10 gm carb)
    Baby Carrots- 5 small
    Pecans- ¼ cup (3.5gm carb)
    Supper 399 calories/30.5gm carb/38gm pro
    Cornish Hen, Roasted- ½ bird
    Northern Beans- ½ cup (18.5gm carb)
    Broccoli Toss
    Small Batch Cornbread- 1 serving (12gm carb)

WEEK 4

22. *Breakfast 210 calories/28gm carb/8gm pro*
    Sweet Potato Breakfast Cup- 1 serving (28gm carb)
    Lunch 633 calories/31gm carb/48gm pro
    Greek Chicken Chopped Salad - 1 serving (11gm carb)
    Parmesan Crisps - 1 serving (1gm carb)
    Honeydew Melon- 1 ¼ cup (19gm carb)

Dinner 652 calories/31gm carb/37gm pro
Steak Kabobs
Roasted Veggies
Potato Skins – 1 serving (12gm carb)
Rye Dinner Roll- 1 medium (19gm carb)

23. *Breakfast 354 calories/31gm carb/16gm pro*
Peanut Butter Sandwich on thin wheat (23 gm carb)
2% Milk- ¾ cup (8 gm carb)
Lunch 293 calories/29gm carb/27gm pro
Pork and Veggie Stir Fry - 1 serving (6gm carb)
Brown Rice- ½ cup (23gm carb)
Dinner 535 calories/31gm carb/40gm pro
Grilled Salmon-5 oz.
Coleslaw – 1 serving (8gm carb)
Baked Sweet Potato- 4 oz. (23gm carb)
Butter or Margarine- 1 Tablespoon

24. *Breakfast 377 calories/31gm carb/22gm pro*
French Toast - 1 serving (23gm carb)
Berry Crush- 1 serving (8gm carb)
Poached Egg- 1
Lunch 429 calories/30gm carb/21gm pro
Pork & Spanish Rice – 1 serving (21gm carb)
Raw Veggie Plate – 1 serving
Ranch Dressing - 2oz. (9gm carb)
Dinner 473 calories/29.5gm carb/28gm pro
Turkey Meatsauce -1 serving (6gm carb)
Whole Wheat Spaghetti- ½ cup (18.5gm carb)
Caesar Salad – 1 serving (5gm carb)

25. *Breakfast 343 calories/32.5gm carb/23gm pro*
Whole Wheat Cooked Cereal- 2/3 cup (22gm carb)
Whole Milk Plain Greek yogurt- 8 oz. (8 gm carb)
Ground Flaxseed- 1 Tablespoon (2.5 gm carb)
Butter or margarine- 1 teaspoon
Lunch 426 calories/29.5gm carb/23gm pro
Pattie Melt w/caramelized onions- 1 serving (14 gm carb)
Ketchup- 1 Tablespoon (4gm carb)
Chopped Watermelon, diced- 1 cup (11.5gm carb)

Dinner 525 calories/29gm carb/32gm carb
Rotisserie Chicken
Roasted Asparagus
Baked Sweet Potato-5 oz. (29gm carb)
Butter or margarine- 1 Tablespoon

26. *Breakfast 252calories/30gm carb/12gm pro*
    Cheesy Eggs
    Mixed Grain Toast-1 slice (11 gm carb)
    Peach- 1 medium (16 gm carb)
    Low sugar jelly- 1 teaspoon (3gm carb)
    Lunch 565 calories/28gm carb/32gm pro
    Taco Salad – 1 serving (26gm carb)
    Sour Cream- ¼ cup (2gm carb)
    Dinner 412 calories/31.5gm carb/33gm pro
    Pineapple Grilled Chicken- 1 serving (6.5gm carb)
    Roasted Green Beans with Onions- 1 serving (2gm carb)
    Wild rice, cooked- 2/3 cup (23gm carb)
    Butter or margarine- 1 Tablespoon

27. *Breakfast 341 calories/27gm carb/15gm pro*
    Veggie Omelet
    English Muffin- Whole Wheat -1 (27gm carb)
    Butter or Margarine- 1 Tablespoon
    Lunch 462 calories/28gm carb/38gm pro
    Turkey Swiss Wrap – 1 serving (28 gm carb)
    Dinner 665 calories/28.5gm/39gm pro
    Grilled Steak- 3 oz.
    Balsamic Mushrooms - 1 serving
    Tossed Salad- medium sized
    Salad Dressing- 1 oz. (5gm carb)
    Potato Skins – 1 servings (12gm carb)
    Watermelon, 1 cup diced (11.5gm carb)

28. *Breakfast 242 calories/29gm carb/15gm pro*
    Oat Bowl- 1 serving (14.5gm carb)
    Raisins- 2 Tablespoons (14.5gm carb)
    Canadian Bacon, grilled- 2 slices
    Lunch 402 calories/32gm carb/14gm pro
    Hummus Lunch Bowl- (32gm Carb)

<u>Dinner 442 calories/30.5gm carb/47gm pro</u>
Beef Chuck Roast- 5 oz.
Carrots, cooked with roast- ½ cup
Lima Beans- ½ cup (17.5gm carb)
Butter or margarine- 1 Tablespoon
Small Batch Cornbread – 1 serving (13gm carb)

APPROX 45GM CARB/MEAL

WEEK 1

1. *Breakfast 360 calories/45.5gm carb/14gm pro*
   Easy Eggs- 1 Serving (.5gm carb)
   Fresh or Frozen (no sugar added) Strawberries- 1 ¼ cup whole berries (15gm carb)
   English Muffin, Whole Wheat- 1 muffin (30gm carb)
   Butter, Light, -1 Tbsp.
   Lunch 650 calories/46.5 gm carb/38gm pro
   Easy Greek Chicken Salad Bowl- 1 serving
   Blueberries- 1 ¼ cup (26gm carb)
   Ranch Salad Dressing 2 Tablespoons- (4.5gm carb)
   Thin Wheat Crackers- 12 (16gm carb)
   Dinner 518 calories/44gm carb/36gm pro
   Grilled BBQ Pork Chop- 1 serving (1gm carb)
   Coleslaw- 3 oz. (8gm carb)
   Deviled Eggs - 2 halves (2gm carb)
   Whole Kernel Corn- ½ cup- (17gm carb)
   Kiwi- 1 (16gm carb)

2. *Breakfast 292 calories/44gm carb/14gm pro*
   Country Egg Sandwich – 1 serving (20 gm carb)
   Tangerines- 2 small (20 gm carb)
   Low Sugar Jelly- ½ Tablespoon (4gm carb)
   Lunch 476 calories/43gm carb/21gm pro
   Flatbread Pizza (28 gm carb)
   Apple w/skin sliced-1 cup (15gm carb)
   Dinner 761 calories/44 gm carb/63gm pro
   Boiled Shrimp- 8 oz. (1 gm carb)
   Tossed Salad -1 cup lettuce/ ½ cup cherry tomatoes
   Ranch Salad Dressing- 3 Tbsp. (2.5gm carb)
   Sunflower Seeds salad topping-1 Tbsp. (2gm carb)
   Thin Wheat Crackers-14- (18.5 gm carb)
   Cantaloupe -1 ½ cup cubes (20 gm carb)

3. *Breakfast 328 calories/46gm carb/15gm pro*
   Greek Yogurt Parfait -1 serving -(31 gm carb)
   Oat Bowl- 1 serving (15gm carb)

Lunch 604 calories/44 gm carb/48gm pro
Greek Chicken Salad – 5.5 oz. (2gm carb) on
   2 Slices Wheat or Rye Bread (30gm carb)
Lettuce- 1/3 cup /Tomato- 1 slice
Light Mayonnaise-1 Tsp.- (2 gm carb)
Baby Carrots- 4 medium-
Low Carb Yogurt- 12 oz. (9 gm carb)
Dinner 560calories/44gm carb/32gm pro
Grilled Sirloin Steak- 3 oz. with Balsamic Mushrooms
Roasted Veggies
Sweet Potato, baked- 5 oz. (30 gm carb)
Pineapple slices, ½ cup (14gm carb)
Margarine or Butter- 1 teaspoon

4. *Breakfast 262 calories/46.5gm carb/13gm pro*
    Oat Bowl- 1 serving (15gm carb)
    Canadian Bacon- 2 slices (.5gm carb)
    Raisins- 2 Tablespoons- (15gm carb)
    Strawberries, sliced- 1 ¼ cup (16gm carb)
    Lunch 669 calories/45gm carb/32gm pro
    Open-Faced Veggie & Beef Burger – 1 serving (14gm carb)
    Sweet Potato Chips-12 chips or 1 oz. (15gm carb)
    Mango, sliced- 2/3 cup (16gm carb)
    Dinner 567 calories/43gm carb/45 gm pro
    Favorite Tacos- 2 tacos (33gm carb)
    Refried Beans- 1/3 cup (10gm carb)

5. *Breakfast 365 calories/43.5gm carb/12gm pro*
    Easy Eggs- 1 serving (.5gm carb)
    Raisin Bread (unfrosted)-2 slices (28gm carb)
    Sliced Strawberries- ½ cup (6gm carb)
    Fruit Spread, 100% fruit-1 Tablespoon (9gm carb)
    Butter or Margarine- 1 Tablespoon
    Lunch 749 calories/43.5gm carb/42gm pro
    Meatballs- 7 medium (10.5 gm carb)
    Whole wheat pasta- ¾ cup (28 gm carb)
    Easy Marinara Sauce- 4 oz. (5gm carb)
    Broccoli Toss – ½ cup
    Parmesan Cheese, grated -2 Tablespoons (.5gm carb)

Dinner 495 calories/44 gm carb/22gm pro
Easy Baked Fish- 3oz.
Baked Sweet Potato-medium 5 oz. - (29gm carb)
Butter or Margarine- 1 Tablespoon
Spinach Salad - 2oz.
Italian Ice- ½ cup (15gm carb)

6. *Breakfast 456 calories/46 gm carb/34gm pro*
   Pork Tenderloin, broiled- 3 oz.
   Oat Bowl- 2 serving (29.5gm carb)
   Raisins- 2 Tablespoons (14 gm carb)
   Flaxseed -ground- 1 Tbsp. -add to oat bowl (2.5gm carb)
   Lunch 653 calories/43 gm carb/37gm pro
   Tomato Soup- 8 oz. (15gm carb)
   Cheese Toast -1 serving (8 gm carb)
   Tossed Salad w/turkey ham,cheese-1 ½ cups
   Salad Dressing- 2 Tablespoons (5 gm carb)
   Apple, fresh- extra small (15 gm carb)
   Dinner 445 calories/43 gm carb/44gm pro
   Turkey Divan- 1 serving (10gm carb)
   Brown Rice 1/3 cup cooked (15gm carb)
   Dark Chocolate-6 gm (4gm carb)
   Peach, fresh- medium (14gm carb)

7. *Breakfast 545 calories/43.5gm carb/33gm pro*
   Breakfast Burrito-1 serving (17gm carb)
   Oat bowl- 1 serving (14.5gm carb)
   Grapes- ¾ cup (12gm carb)
   Lunch 399 calories/44.5 gm carb/21gm pro
   Tuna Salad- ½ cup (9.5gm carb) with celery, baby carrots, tomato slices
   Thin Wheat Crackers-16 (22gm carb)
   Tomato, Fresh- 2 slices
   Cantaloupe- 1 cup, diced (13 gm carb)
   Dinner 399 calories/44 gm carb/43gm pro
   Herb-Roasted Chicken & Veggies – 1 serving
   Whole Kernel Corn- ½ cup (15gm carb)
   Canned Peaches, Juice Pack- ½ cup (15gm carb)
   Cranberry Sauce- 2 Tablespoons (14gm carb)

WEEK 2

8. *Breakfast 288 calories/43gm carb/13gm pro*
   Oatmeal Banana Smoothie (28gm carb)
   Raisin Bread, unfrosted- 1 slice (14gm carb)
   Almonds, roasted- 1 Tablespoons (1gm carb)
   Lunch 563 calories/44.5gm carb/48gm pro
   Greek Chicken Sandwich (22 gm carb)
   Vegetable Soup- 1 cup (8gm carb)
   Wheat Crackers- 10 (14.5gm carb)
   Dinner 523 calories/45.5gm carb/33gm pro
   Balsamic Pork Tenderloin- 4.5gm serving (1.5gm carb)
   Small Baked Sweet Potato- 5 oz. (29gm Carb)
   Butter or Margarine- 1 Tablespoon
   Spinach Salad
   Apple with skin, sliced- 1 cup (15gm carb)

9. *Breakfast 338 calories/43.5gm carb/13gm pro*
   English muffin-1 (28gm carb)
   Butter or Margarine- 1 Tablespoon
   Poached Egg-1
   Blueberries- ¾ cup (15.5gm carb)
   Lunch 806 calories/46gm carb/53 gm pro
   Steak Kabobs- 10 oz.
   Tossed Salad w/ham, turkey, cheese- 1 ½ cup
   Ranch Dressing- 2 Tablespoons (1.5gm carb)
   Wild Rice, cooked- 1 cup (35gm carb)
   Plums, sliced- ½ cup (9.5 gm carb)
   Dinner 325 calories/45gm carb/16gm pro
   Eggplant Parm- 1 serving (11.5gm carb)
   Whole Wheat Pasta- ½ cup (18.5gm carb)
   Olives, Black, chopped- 3 Tablespoons
   Mandarin Oranges – ¾ cup (15gm carb)

10. *Breakfast 457 calories/46 gm carb/23gm pro*
    French Toast – 1 serving (23gm carb)
    Berry Crush- 1 serving (8gm carb)
    Bacon- 2 slices
    Butter- 1 Tablespoon
    Nectarine, small-1 (15gm carb)

Lunch   644 calories/45.5gm carb/40 gm pro
Chef's Salad w/cheese, egg, turkey, ham, lettuce, tomato
Grapes, 17 small (15gm carb)
Whole wheat croutons- 2/3 cup (14 gm carb)
Salad Dressing, Light-3 Tablespoons (3gm carb)
Thin Wheat Crackers- 10 (13.5 gm carb)
Dinner   512 calories/43gm carb/33gm pro
Roast Beef Sandwich on thin whole wheat bread (20 gm carb)
with lettuce & tomato
Honey mustard dressing- 2 Tablespoons (8gm carb)
Gazpacho Soup- 1 cup
Potato Salad-4 oz. (15gm carb)

11. *Breakfast   481 calories/44gm carb/21gm pro*
    Oat Bowl- 1 serving (15gm carb)
    Ham, Egg and Veggie Roll Up -1 serving
    Raisins-2 Tablespoons (14gm carb)
    Whole Wheat Toast- 1 slice (15gm carb)
    Butter or Margarine- 1 Tablespoon
    Lunch   715 calories/45gm carb/63gm pro
    Greek Chicken Salad Stuffed Pita – 2 serving (26 gm carb)
    Honeydew Melon, cubed- 1 ¼ cup (19 gm carb)
    Dinner   604 calories/44.5 gm carb/38gm pro
    Fried Rice – 1 serving (24.5gm carb)
    Cashews- .75oz. or 8-10 (6gm carb)
    Sweet & Sour Sauce- 2 Tablespoons (14gm carb)

12. *Breakfast   468 calories/43gm carb/27gm pro*
    Raisin bread, unfrosted- 2 slices (30 gm carb)
    Eggs in Ham Cups- 1 serving
    2% milk- 1 cup (12gm carb)
    Cream Cheese- 2 Tablespoons (1gm carb)
    Lunch 303 calories/43gm carb/17gm pro
    Crunchy Fish Tacos with Caribbean Slaw - 1 serving (28gm carb)
    Banana Ice Cream- 1 serving (15gm carb)

Dinner 732 calories/44gm carb/28gm pro
Chili with beans- ¾ cup (24gm carb)
Sour Cream- 2 Tablespoons (2gm carb)
Cheddar Cheese, shredded- 2 oz. (1gm carb)
Side Salad- 3 oz.
Ranch Dressing- 2 Tablespoons (2gm carb)
Chocolate Berries- 1 serving (15gm carb)

13. *Breakfast 398 calories/45.5gm carb/12 gm pro*
    Apple-Nut Sandwich – 1 serving (31 gm carb)
    Oat Bowl- 1 serving (14.5gm carb)
    Lunch 693 calories/45gm carb/41gm pro
    Turkey Swiss Wrap (25gm carb)
    Avocado Cubed, 1/3 cup (4 gm carb)
    Sweet Potato Chips – 1 oz. (16gm carb)
    Dinner 576 calories/45gm carb/45gm pro
    Spinach Salad with Grilled Shrimp- 5 oz.
    Thin Wheat Crackers- 11 (15gm carb)
    Strawberries, sliced- 1 1/3 cup (16.5gm carb)
    Whipped Cream- 2 Tablespoons (1gm carb)
    Dark Chocolate Bar, miniature- 3 bars (12.5gm carb)

14. *Breakfast 534 calories/46.5gm carb/33gm pro*
    Eggs Benedict – 2 serving (34 gm carb)
    Fresh Peach, small (12.5 gm carb)
    Lunch 491 calories/46.5gm carb/27 gm pro
    Tortilla Pizza -2 serving (46.5gm carb)
    Dinner 689 calories/44gm carb/44gm pro
    Salmon Pattie- 2 servings (12gm carb)
    Coleslaw - 1 serving (8gm carb)
    Potato Skins- 1 serving (12gm carb)
    Mango, sliced- ½ cup (12gm carb)

WEEK 3

15. *Breakfast 422 calories/46gm carb/28gm pro*
    Breakfast Banana Split- 1 serving (31gm carb)
    High Protein Oatmeal- 1 serving (15gm carb)

Lunch 467 calories/43gm carb/28gm pro
Red & White Chicken Chili- 1 serving (30gm carb)
Small Batch Cornbread- 1 serving (13gm carb)
Sour Cream- 2 Tablespoons (1gm carb)
Cheddar Cheese, shredded- 1 oz.
Dinner 494 calories/44.5gm carb/40gm pro
Jerk Chicken
Caribbean Coleslaw- 1 serving
Roasted Sweet Potatoes- 1 cup (26gm carb)
Mango, diced- ¾ cup (18.5gm carb)
Butter or margarine- 1 Tablespoon

16. *Breakfast 359 calories/44.5gm carb/16gm pro*
    Oat Bowl with Cinnamon- 1 serving (14.5 gm carb)
    Large Apple- sliced (30gm carb)
    Boiled Egg-2
    Lunch 662 calories/43gm carb/67gm pro
    Greek Chicken Wrap – 2 servings (27gm carb)
    Blueberries- ¾ cup (16gm carb)
    Dinner 475 calories/43gm carb/28gm pro
    Lighter Lasagna Caprese- 1.5 servings (43gm carb)

17. *Breakfast 480 calories/43.5gm carb/36gm pro*
    Pork Tenderloin, grilled – 3 oz.
    Oat Bowl- 1 serving (14.5gm carb)
    Cinnamon Toast- 1 serving (20gm carb)
    Small Banana- ½ (9 gm carb)
    Lunch 779 calories/45.5gm carb/60gm pro
    Cobb Salad Platter – 1 serving (3gm carb)
    Wheat Croutons- ¾ cup (16gm carb)
    Ranch Salad Dressing -2 Tablespoons (5gm carb)
    Crackers, Multigrain, 4 crackers (9.5gm carb)
    Grapes- ¾ cup (12gm carb)
    Dinner 415 calories/44.5gm carb/26gm pro
    Pork Tenderloin with Apples -1 serving (10.5gm carb)
    Roasted Green Beans with Onions- 1 cup
    Sweet Potato, baked- 1 medium-3.5oz. (20gm carb)
    Butter or Margarine- 1 Tablespoon
    Wheat Dinner roll- 1 (14 gm carb)

18. *Breakfast 467 calories/45 gm carb/15gm pro*
    Egg Baked in Avocado Cups – 1 serving (9gm carb)
    Whole Wheat English Muffin- 1 (28gm carb)
    Grapes- ½ cup (8gm carb)
    Butter or Margarine- 1 Tablespoon
    Lunch 713 calories/45.5gm carb/30gm pro
    Beef & Vegetable Soup -10 oz. (14gm carb)
    Cheese Toast- 2 serving (16gm carb)
    Side Salad- 6 oz.
    Bacon & Tomato Salad Dressing- 2 Tablespoons (.5gm carb)
    Chocolate Berries- 1 serving (15gm carb)
    Dinner 423 calories/45.5gm carb/29gm pro
    Veracruz Style Snapper – 1 serving
    Lima Beans- ¾ cup (30.5gm carb)
    Brown Rice- 1/3 cup (15gm carb)

19. *Breakfast 404 calories/44gm carb/15gm pro*
    High Protein Oatmeal - 2 servings (30gm carb)
    Raisins- 2 Tablespoons (14gm carb)
    Butter or Margarine- 1 Tablespoon
    Lunch 385 calories/43gm carb/28gm pro
    Grilled Shrimp Wrap – 1 serving (28gm carb)
    Strawberries, sliced- 1 ¼ cup (15gm carb)
    Dinner 467calories/44gm carb/40gm pro
    Oven Baked BBQ Ribs -1 serving
    Baked Beans, low sugar- ½ cup (22gm carb)
    Butter or Margarine- 1 Tablespoon
    Coleslaw – 1 serving (8gm carb)
    Watermelon, diced- 1 ¼ cup (14gm carb)

20. *Breakfast 455 calories/44.5gm carb/18gm pro*
    5 Grain Cooked Cereal or oatmeal- 1 cup (30gm carb)
    2 Tablespoons Raisins (14.5gm carb)
    Cheesy Eggs- 1 serving
    Bacon, Baked- 2 strips
    Butter- 1 Tablespoon
    Lunch 650 calories/43 gm carb/38gm pro
    Chicken and Veggie Stir Fry -1 serving
    Sweet & Sour Sauce- 1 Tablespoon (7 gm carb)
    Brown Rice- 2/3 cup (30gm carb)
    Peanuts- 1 ounce (6gm carb)

Dinner 460 calories/45gm carb/28gm pro
Beef & Bean Burrito-1 (45gm carb)

21. *Breakfast 396 calories/46.5gm carb/18gm pro*
    English Muffin Stack – 1 serving (26gm carb)
    Low Sugar Jelly- 2 teaspoons (5.5gm carb)
    Blueberries- ¾ cup (15gm carb)
    Lunch 694 calories/44.5gm carb/33gm pro
    Tuna Salad Stuffed Tomato- 6oz. (16gm carb)
    Thin Wheat Crackers-8 (10 gm carb)
    Baby Carrots- 5 small
    Pecans- ¼ cup (3.5gm carb)
    Bananas- ½ cup (15gm carb)
    Supper 565 calories/43.5gm carb/45gm pro
    Cornish Hen, Roasted- ½ bird
    Northern Beans- ½ cup (18.5gm carb)
    Broccoli Toss
    Small Batch Cornbread- 2 servings (25gm carb)

WEEK 4

22. *Breakfast 282 calories/45gm carb/9gm pro*
    Sweet Potato Breakfast Cup- 1 serving (28gm carb)
    Kiwi, sliced- 2/3 cups (17gm carb)
    Lunch 837 calories/47gm carb/50gm pro
    Greek Chicken Chopped Salad - 1 serving (11gm carb)
    Cheese Toast- 2 servings (17gm carb)
    Honeydew Melon- 1 ¼ cup (19gm carb)
    Dinner 905 calories/46gm carb/50gm pro
    Steak Kabobs
    Roasted Veggies
    Potato Skins – 2 serving (24gm carb)
    Rye Dinner Roll- 1 large (22gm carb)

23. *Breakfast 430 calories/45gm carb/19gm pro*
    Peanut Butter Sandwich on wheat bread- 2 slices (37 gm carb)
    ¾ cup milk (8 gm carb)
    Lunch 384 calories/44gm carb/29gm pro
    Pork and Veggie Stir Fry - 1 serving (6gm carb)
    Brown Rice- ½ cup (23gm carb)
    Pineapple chunks- ½ cup (15gm carb)

Dinner 570 calories/46gm carb/41gm pro
Grilled Salmon-5 oz.
Coleslaw – 1 serving (8gm carb)
Baked Sweet Potato- 4 oz. (23gm carb)
Butter or Margarine- 1 Tablespoon
Banana Ice Cream- 1 serving (15gm carb)

24. *Breakfast 476 calories/44gm carb/29gm pro*
French Toast - 1 serving (23gm carb)
Berry Crush- 1 serving (8gm carb)
Poached Egg- 1
Greek Yogurt – 4 oz. (14 gm carb)
Lunch 529 calories/46gm carb/27gm pro
Pork & Spanish Rice – 1 serving (21gm carb)
Refried Beans- ½ cup (16gm carb)
Raw Veggie Plate – 1 serving
Ranch Dressing - 2oz. (9gm carb)
Dinner 590 calories/44.5gm carb/32gm pro
Turkey Meatsauce -1 serving (6gm carb)
Whole Wheat Spaghetti- ½ cup (18.5gm carb)
Caesar Salad – 1 serving (5gm carb)
Whole wheat Breadstick or Roll-1 (15gm carb)

25. *Breakfast 404 calories/47.5gm carb/24 gm pro*
Whole Wheat Cooked Cereal- 2/3 cup (22gm carb)
Whole Milk Plain Greek yogurt- 8 oz. (8 gm carb)
Ground Flaxseed- 1 Tablespoon (2.5 gm carb)
Butter or Margarine- 1 teaspoon
Banana- ½ large (15gm carb)
Lunch 577 calories/45.5gm carb/24gm pro
Pattie Melt w/ caramelized onions- 1 serving (14 gm carb)
Ketchup- 1 Tablespoon (4gm carb)
Chopped Watermelon, diced- 1 cup (11.5gm carb)
Sweet potato chips- 1 oz. (16gm carb)
Dinner 482 calories/44 gm carb/33gm carb
Rotisserie Chicken - 1 serving
Roasted Asparagus -1 serving
Baked Sweet Potato-5 oz. (29gm carb)
Butter or margarine- 1 Tablespoon
Chocolate Berries- 1 serving (15gm carb)

26. *Breakfast 321 calories/43gm carb/15gm pro*
   Cheesy Eggs
   Mixed Grain Toast-2 slices (24gm carb)
   Peach- 1 medium (16 gm carb)
   Low sugar jelly- 1 teaspoon (3gm carb)
   Lunch 633 calories/44 gm carb/34gm pro
   Taco Salad – 1 serving (26gm carb)
   Sour Cream- ¼ cup (2gm carb)
   Nectarine, large- 1 (16gm carb)
   Dinner 537 calories/46.5gm carb/34gm pro
   Pineapple Grilled Chicken- 1 serving (6.5gm carb)
   Roasted Green Beans with Onions- 1 serving (2gm carb)
   Wild rice, cooked- 2/3 cup (23gm carb)
   Butter or margarine- 1 Tablespoon
   Dark Chocolate- 4 pieces-24gm (15gm carb)

27. *Breakfast 402 calories/42gm carb/16gm pro*
   Veggie Omelet
   English Muffin- Whole Wheat -1 (27gm carb)
   Butter or Margarine- 1 Tablespoon
   Honeydew Melon. Diced- 1 cup (15gm carb)
   Lunch 521 calories/42gm carb/40gm pro
   Turkey Swiss Wrap – 1 serving (28 gm carb)
   Peach, medium-1 (14gm carb)
   Dinner 740 calories/43.5gm/42gm pro
   Grilled Steak- 3 oz.
   Balsamic Mushrooms - 1 serving
   Tossed Salad- medium sized
   Salad Dressing- 1 oz. (5gm carb)
   Potato Skins – 1 servings (12gm carb)
   Wheat roll, small-1 (15gm carb)
   Watermelon, 1 cup diced (11.5gm carb)

28. *Breakfast 342 calories/43.5gm carb/19gm pro*
   Oat Bowl- 2 servings (29gm carb)
   Raisins- 2 Tablespoons (14.5gm carb)
   Canadian Bacon, grilled- 2 slices

<u>Lunch 457 calories/46 gm carb/15gm pro</u>
<u>Hummus Lunch Bowl</u>- (32gm Carb)
<u>Blueberries</u>- 2/3 cup (14gm carb)
<u>Dinner 541 calories/45 gm carb/48gm pro</u>
Beef Chuck Roast- 5 oz.
Carrots, cooked with roast- ½ cup
Lima Beans- ½ cup (17.5gm carb)
Butter or margarine- 1 Tablespoon
Small Batch Cornbread – 1 serving (13gm carb)
<u>Baked Pear</u>- 1 serving (14.5 gm carb)

APPROX 60GM CARB/MEAL

WEEK 1

1. ***Breakfast 427 calories/60.5gm carb/17gm pro***
   Easy Eggs- 1 Serving (.5gm carb)
   Fresh or Frozen (no sugar added) Strawberries- 1 ¼ cup whole berries (15gm carb)
   English Muffin, Whole Wheat- 1 ½ muffin (45gm carb)
   Butter, Light, -1 Tbsp.
   Lunch 741 calories/59.5 gm carb/40gm pro
   Easy Greek Chicken Salad Bowl- 1 serving
   Blueberries- 1 ¼ cup (26 gm carb)
   Ranch Salad Dressing 2 Tablespoons- (4.5gm carb)
   Thin Wheat Crackers- 22 (29 gm carb)
   Dinner 583 calories/61gm carb/38gm pro
   Grilled BBQ Pork Chop- 1 serving (1gm carb)
   Coleslaw- 3 oz. (8gm carb)
   Deviled Eggs - 2 halves (2gm carb)
   Whole Kernel Corn- ½ cup- (17gm carb)
   Kiwi, sliced- 1.25 cup (33gm carb)

2. ***Breakfast 470 calories/60gm carb/26gm pro***
   Country Egg Sandwich – 2 serving (40 gm carb)
   Tangerines- 2 small (20 gm carb)
   Lunch 838 calories/61gm carb/42gm pro
   Flatbread Pizza (61 gm carb)
   Dinner 806 calories/58.5gm carb/66gm pro
   Boiled Shrimp- 8 oz. (1 gm carb)
   Tossed Salad -1 cup lettuce/ ½ cup cherry tomatoes
   Ranch Salad Dressing- 3 Tbsp. (2.5gm carb)
   Sunflower Seeds salad topping-1 Tbsp. (2gm carb)
   Whole Wheat Roll- 1 (33 gm carb)
   Cantaloupe -1 ½ cup cubes (20 gm carb)

3. ***Breakfast 428 calories/60 gm carb/18gm pro***
   Greek Yogurt Parfait -1 serving -(31 gm carb)
   Oat Bowl- 2 serving (29gm carb)

Lunch 667 calories/58 gm carb/48gm pro
Greek Chicken Salad – 5.5 oz. (2gm carb) on
  2 Slices Wheat or Rye Bread (30gm carb)
Lettuce- 1/3 cup /Tomato- 1 slice
Light Mayonnaise-1 Tsp.- (2 gm carb)
Baby Carrots- 4 medium-
Low Carb Yogurt- 12 oz. (9 gm carb)
Grapes- 1 cup (15gm carb)
Dinner 595calories/59gm carb/33gm pro
Grilled Sirloin Steak- 3 oz. with Balsamic Mushrooms
Roasted Veggies
Sweet Potato, baked- 5 oz. (30 gm carb)
Pineapple, fresh, chunks, 1 1/3 cup (29gm carb)
Margarine or Butter- 1 teaspoon

4. *Breakfast 362 calories/61.5gm carb/16gm pro*
Oat Bowl- 2 servings (30gm carb)
Canadian Bacon- 2 slices (.5gm carb)
Raisins- 2 Tablespoons- (15gm carb)
Strawberries, sliced- 1 ¼ cup (16gm carb)
Lunch 819 calories/60gm carb/34gm pro
Open-Faced Veggie & Beef Burger – 1 serving (14gm carb)
Sweet Potato Chips-24 chips or 2 oz. (30gm carb)
Mango, sliced- 2/3 cup (16gm carb)
Dinner 820 calories/60gm carb/65 gm pro
Favorite Tacos- 3 tacos (50gm carb)
Refried Beans- 1/3 cup (10gm carb)

5. *Breakfast 419 calories/57.5gm carb/13gm pro*
Easy Eggs- 1 serving (.5gm carb)
Raisin Bread (unfrosted)-2 slices (28gm carb)
Sliced Strawberries-1 ½ cup (20gm carb)
Fruit Spread, 100% fruit-1 Tablespoon (9gm carb)
Butter or Margarine- 1 Tablespoon
Lunch 902 calories/60 gm carb/43gm pro
Meatballs- 7 medium (10.5 gm carb)
Whole wheat pasta- 2/3 cup (24 gm carb)
Easy Marinara Sauce- 4 oz. (5gm carb)
Broccoli Toss – ½ cup
Parmesan Cheese, grated -2 Tablespoons (.5gm carb)
Berries with Coconut and Whipped Cream- 1 serving (20gm carb)

Dinner 599 calories/57 gm carb/25gm pro
Easy Baked Fish- 3oz.
Baked Sweet Potato-medium 5 oz. - (29gm carb)
Small Batch Cornbread-1 serving (13gm carb)
Butter or Margarine- 1 Tablespoon
Spinach Salad - 2oz.
Italian Ice- ½ cup (15gm carb)

6. *Breakfast 571 calories/62 gm carb/37gm pro*
   Pork Tenderloin, broiled- 3 oz.
   Oat Bowl- 2 serving (29.5gm carb)
   Raisins- 2 Tablespoons (14 gm carb)
   Flaxseed -ground- 1 Tbsp. -add to oat bowl (2.5gm carb)
   Wheat Bread, toasted- 1 slice (16gm carb)
   Butter or Margarine- 1 teaspoon
   Lunch 716 calories/58gm carb/38gm pro
   8 oz. Tomato Soup- (15gm carb)
   Cheese Toast -1 serving (8 gm carb)
   Tossed Salad w/turkey ham,cheese-1 ½ cups
   Salad Dressing- 2 Tablespoons (5 gm carb)
   Apple, fresh- large (30 gm carb)
   Dinner 517 calories/58 gm carb/46gm pro
   Turkey Divan- 1 serving (10gm carb)
   Brown Rice 2/3 cup cooked (30gm carb)
   Dark Chocolate-6 gm (4gm carb)
   Peach, fresh- medium (14gm carb)

7. *Breakfast 545 calories/58 gm carb/33gm pro*
   Breakfast Burrito-1 serving (17gm carb)
   Oat bowl- 2 servings (29 gm carb)
   Grapes- ¾ cup (12gm carb)
   Lunch 460 calories/59.5 gm carb/22gm pro
   Tuna Salad- ½ cup (9.5gm carb) with celery, baby carrots, tomato slices
   Thin Wheat Crackers-16 (22gm carb)
   Tomato, Fresh- 2 slices
   Cantaloupe- 1 cup, diced (13 gm carb)
   Banana Ice Cream, 1 serving (15gm carb)

Dinner 465 calories/59 gm carb/47gm pro
<u>Herb-Roasted Chicken & Veggies</u> – 1 serving
Whole Kernel Corn- ½ cup (15gm carb)
Peas, Green- ½ cup (15gm carb)
Canned Peaches, Juice Pack- ½ cup (15gm carb)
Cranberry Sauce- 2 Tablespoons (14gm carb)

WEEK 2

8. *Breakfast 359 calories/57gm carb/15gm pro*
   <u>Oatmeal Banana Smoothie</u> (28gm carb)
   Raisin Bread, unfrosted- 2 slice (28gm carb)
   <u>Almonds, roasted</u>- 1 Tablespoons (1gm carb)
   Lunch 667 calories/60.5gm carb/48gm pro
   <u>Greek Chicken Sandwich</u> (22 gm carb)
   Cream of Tomato Soup- 1 cup (24gm carb)
   Wheat Crackers- 10 (14.5gm carb)
   Dinner 667 calories/59.5gm carb/37gm pro
   <u>Balsamic Pork Tenderloin</u>- 4.5gm serving (1.5gm carb)
   Small Baked Sweet Potato- 5 oz. (29gm Carb)
   Butter or Margarine- 1 Tablespoon
   <u>Spinach Salad</u>
   <u>Baked Apple</u>- 1 serving (29gm carb)

9. *Breakfast 438 calories/58gm carb/17gm pro*
   Oat Bowl- 1 serving (14.5)
   English muffin-1 (28gm carb)
   Butter or Margarine- 1 Tablespoon
   Poached Egg-1
   Blueberries- ¾ cup (15.5gm carb)
   Lunch 866 calories/59.5gm carb/56 gm pro
   <u>Steak Kabobs</u>- 10 oz.
   Tossed Salad w/ham, turkey, cheese- 1 ½ cup
   Ranch Dressing- 1 Tablespoon (<1gm carb)
   Wild Rice, cooked- 1 cup (35gm carb)
   Plums, sliced- ½ cup (9.5 gm carb)
   Ice Cream, No Sugar Added- ½ cup (15gm carb)

Dinner 578 calories/61.5gm carb/27gm pro
Eggplant Parm- 1 serving (11.5gm carb)
Whole Wheat Pasta- 2/3 cup (25gm carb)
Caesar Salad- 1 serving (5gm carb)
Mandarin Oranges – 1 cup (20gm carb)

10. *Breakfast 520 calories/61 gm carb/24gm pro*
    French Toast – 1 serving (23gm carb)
    Berry Crush- 1 serving (8gm carb)
    Bacon- 2 slices
    Butter- 1 Tablespoon
    Nectarine, small-2 (30gm carb)
    Lunch   999 calories/62.5gm carb/57 gm pro
    Chef's Salad w/ cheese, egg, turkey, ham, lettuce, tomato
    Grapes, 17 small (15gm carb)
    Whole wheat croutons- 2/3 cup (14 gm carb)
    Salad Dressing, Light-3 Tablespoons (3gm carb)
    Thin Wheat Crackers- 10 (13.5 gm carb)
    Cheese Toast- 2 servings (17gm carb)
    Dinner   572 calories/58gm carb/34gm pro
    Roast Beef Sandwich on thin whole wheat bread (20 gm carb)
    with lettuce & tomato
    Honey mustard dressing- 2 Tablespoons (8gm carb)
    Gazpacho Soup- 1 cup
    Potato Salad-4 oz. (15gm carb)
    Banana Ice Cream- 1 serving (15gm carb)

11. *Breakfast   573 calories/59gm carb/23gm pro*
    Oat Bowl- 1 serving (15gm carb)
    Ham, Egg and Veggie Roll Up -1 serving
    Raisins-2 Tablespoons (14gm carb)
    Whole Wheat Toast- 2 slice (30gm carb)
    Butter or Margarine- 1 Tablespoon
    Lunch 866 calories/61gm carb/64gm pro
    Greek Chicken Salad Stuffed Pita – 2 serving (26 gm carb)
    1 ¼ cup cubed honeydew (19 gm carb)
    Sweet Potato Chips- 1 oz. (16gm carb)

Dinner   712 calories/61.5 gm carb/42gm pro
Fried Rice – 1 serving (24.5gm carb)
Cashews- .75 oz. or 8-10 (6gm carb)
Egg Roll- 2.5"diameter (17gm carb)
Sweet & Sour Sauce- 2 Tablespoons (14gm carb)

12. *Breakfast   529 calories/58gm carb/27gm pro*
    Raisin bread, unfrosted- 2 slices (30 gm carb)
    Eggs in Ham Cups- 1 serving
    2% milk- 1 cup (12gm carb)
    Cream Cheese- 2 Tablespoons (1gm carb)
    Honeydew Melon, diced -1 cup (15gm carb)
    Lunch   364 calories/58gm carb/18gm pro
    Crunchy Fish Tacos with Caribbean Slaw - 1 serving (28gm carb)
    Banana Ice Cream- 2 servings (30gm carb)
    Dinner 838 calories/59gm carb/29gm pro
    Chili with beans- ¾ cup (24gm carb)
    Sour Cream- 2 Tablespoons (2gm carb)
    Cheddar Cheese, shredded- 2 oz. (1gm carb)
    Side Salad- 3 oz.
    Ranch Dressing- 2 Tablespoons (2gm carb)
    Chocolate Berries- 2 servings (30gm carb)

13. *Breakfast 498 calories/60gm carb/15gm pro*
    Apple-Nut Sandwich – 1 serving (31 gm carb)
    Oat Bowl- 2 serving (29gm carb)
    Lunch 844 calories/61gm carb/41gm pro
    Turkey Swiss Wrap (25gm carb)
    Avocado Cubed, 1/3 cup (4 gm carb)
    Sweet Potato Chips – 2 oz. (32gm carb)
    Dinner 687 calories/57.5gm carb/47gm pro
    Spinach Salad with Grilled Shrimp- 5 oz.
    Thin Wheat Crackers- 15 (20gm carb)
    Strawberries, sliced- 1 1/3 cup (16.5gm carb)
    Whipped Cream- 2 Tablespoons (1gm carb)
    Dark Chocolate Bar, miniature- 5 bars (20gm carb)

14. *Breakfast 584 calories/59gm carb/34gm pro*
    Eggs Benedict – 2 serving (34 gm carb)
    Fresh Peach, small-2 (25 gm carb)

Lunch 577 calories/59.5gm carb/29 gm pro
Tortilla Pizza -2 serving (46.5gm carb)
Summer Corn Salad- 5 oz. (13gm carb)
Dinner 939 calories/60gm carb/56gm pro
Salmon Pattie- 2 servings (12gm carb)
Coleslaw - 1 serving (8gm carb)
Potato Skins- 2 serving (24gm carb)
Mango, sliced- 2/3 cup (16gm carb)

WEEK 3

15. *Breakfast 562 calories/61gm carb/35gm pro*
    Breakfast Banana Split- 1 serving (31gm carb)
    High Protein Oatmeal- 2 servings (30gm carb)
    Lunch 571 calories/56gm carb/31gm pro
    Red & White Chicken Chili- 1 serving (30gm carb)
    Small Batch Cornbread- 2 serving (26gm carb)
    Sour Cream- 2 Tablespoons (1gm carb)
    Cheddar Cheese, shredded- 1 oz.
    Dinner 569 calories/59.5gm carb/43gm pro
    Jerk Chicken
    Caribbean Coleslaw- 1 serving
    Roasted Sweet Potatoes- 1 cup (26gm carb)
    Mango, diced- ¾ cup (18.5gm carb)
    Butter or margarine- 1 Tablespoon
    Whole Wheat Roll- 1 oz. (15gm carb)

16. *Breakfast 460 calories/59gm carb/20gm pro*
    Oat Bowl with Cinnamon- 2 servings (29 gm carb)
    Large Apple- sliced (30gm carb)
    Boiled Egg-2
    Lunch 798 calories/61gm carb/68gm pro
    Greek Chicken Wrap – 2 servings (27gm carb)
    Blueberry Crisp- 2 serving (34gm carb)
    Dinner 497 calories/57gm carb/25gm pro
    Lighter Lasagna Caprese- 1 servings (28gm carb)
    English Peas- ½ cup (12gm carb)
    Whole Wheat Bread, toasted- 1 slice (17gm carb)
    Butter or margarine- 1 teaspoon

17. *Breakfast 580 calories/58gm carb/39gm pro*
    Pork Tenderloin, grilled – 3 oz.
    Oat Bowl- 2 servings (29gm carb)
    Cinnamon Toast- 1 serving (20gm carb)
    Small Banana- ½ (9 gm carb)
    Lunch 880 calories/58gm carb/62gm pro
    Cobb Salad Platter – 1 serving (3gm carb)
    Wheat Croutons- ¾ cup (16gm carb)
    Ranch Salad Dressing -2 Tablespoons (5gm carb)
    Crackers, Multigrain, 4 crackers (9.5gm carb)
    Grapes- ¾ cup (12gm carb)
    Broccoli Cheese Soup- 1 cup (13gm carb)
    Dinner 569 calories/60gm carb/46gm pro
    Pork Tenderloin with Apples -2 servings (22gm carb)
    Roasted Green Beans with Onions- 1 cup
    Sweet Potato, baked- 1 medium-4oz. (24gm carb)
    Butter or Margarine- 1 Tablespoon
    Wheat Dinner roll- 1 (14 gm carb)

18. *Breakfast 549 calories/60 gm carb/18gm pro*
    Egg Baked in Avocado Cups – 1 serving (9gm carb)
    Whole Wheat English Muffin- 1.5 (40gm carb)
    Grapes- ¾ cup (11gm carb)
    Butter or Margarine- 1 Tablespoon
    Lunch 820 calories/60.5gm carb/31gm pro
    Beef & Vegetable Soup -10 oz. (14gm carb)
    Cheese Toast- 2 serving (16gm carb)
    Side Salad- 6 oz.
    Bacon & Tomato Salad Dressing- 2 Tablespoons (.5gm carb)
    Chocolate Berries- 2 servings (30gm carb)
    Dinner 495 calories/60.5gm carb/31gm pro
    Veracruz Style Snapper – 1 serving
    Lima Beans- ¾ cup (30.5gm carb)
    Brown Rice- 2/3 cup (30gm carb)

19. *Breakfast 496 calories/60gm carb/18gm pro*
    High Protein Oatmeal - 2 servings (30gm carb)
    Raisins- 2 Tablespoons (14gm carb)
    Butter or Margarine- 1 Tablespoon
    Whole Wheat Toast- 1 slice (16gm carb)

Lunch 656 calories/60gm carb/53gm pro
Grilled Shrimp Wrap – 2 servings (56gm carb)
Strawberries, sliced- 1/3 cup (4gm carb)
Dinner 569 calories/58gm carb/42gm pro
Oven Baked BBQ Ribs -1 serving
Baked Beans, low sugar- ½ cup (22gm carb)
Butter or Margarine- 1 Tablespoon
Coleslaw 2 serving (16gm carb)
Watermelon, diced- 1 ¾ cup (20gm carb)

20. *Breakfast 547 calories/60.5gm carb/21gm pro*
5 Grain Cooked Cereal or oatmeal- 1 cup (30gm carb)
2 Tablespoons Raisins (14.5gm carb)
Whole Wheat Toast- 1 slice (16gm carb)
Cheesy Eggs- 1 serving
Bacon, Baked- 2 strips
Butter- 1 Tablespoon
Lunch 817 calories/63 gm carb/40gm pro
Chicken and Veggie Stir Fry -1 serving
Sweet & Sour Sauce- 1 Tablespoon (7 gm carb)
Brown Rice- 2/3 cup (30gm carb)
Peanuts- 1 ounce (6gm carb)
Berries with Coconut and Whipped Cream- 1 serving (20gm carb)
Dinner 618 calories/59gm carb/31gm pro
Beef & Bean Burrito- 1 (45gm carb)
Salsa- ½ cup (8 gm carb)
Avocado, diced- ½ cup (6gm carb)

21. *Breakfast 645 calories/57.5gm carb/35gm pro*
English Muffin Stack – 2 servings (52gm carb)
Low Sugar Jelly- 2 teaspoons (5.5gm carb)
Lunch 785 calories/59.5gm carb/35gm pro
Tuna Salad Stuffed Tomato- 6oz. (16gm carb)
Thin Wheat Crackers-18 (25 gm carb)
Baby Carrots- 5 small
Pecans- ¼ cup (3.5gm carb)
Bananas- ½ cup (15gm carb)

Supper 668 calories/61gm carb/48gm pro
Cornish Hen, Roasted- ½ hen
Northern Beans- 2/3 cup (24gm carb)
Broccoli Toss
Small Batch Cornbread- 3 servings (37gm carb)

WEEK 4

22. *Breakfast 420 calories/57 gm carb/15gm pro*
    Sweet Potato Breakfast Cup- 2 serving (57gm carb)
    Lunch 673 calories/59gm carb/42gm pro
    Greek Chicken Chopped Salad - 1 serving (11gm carb)
    Black Bean Soup- 6 oz. (25gm carb)
    Honeydew Melon- 1 ½ cup (23gm carb)
    Dinner 984 calories/60gm carb/51gm pro
    Steak Kabobs
    Roasted Veggies
    Potato Skins – 2 serving (24gm carb)
    Rye Dinner Roll- 1 medium (19gm carb)
    Blueberry Crisp- 1 serving (17gm carb)

23. *Breakfast 503 calories/58gm carb/21gm pro*
    Peanut Butter (2 Tbsp.) Sandwich on 2 slices wheat bread-(37 gm carb)
    Milk- 8 oz. (10 gm carb)
    Banana, sliced- 1/3 cup (11gm carb)
    Lunch 436 calories/58gm carb/29gm pro
    Pork and Veggie Stir Fry - 1 serving (6gm carb)
    Brown Rice- ½ cup (23gm carb)
    Sweet & Sour Sauce- 2 Tbsp. (14gm carb)
    Pineapple chunks- ½ cup (15gm carb)
    Dinner 630 calories/61gm carb/41gm pro
    Grilled Salmon-5 oz.
    Coleslaw – 1 serving (8gm carb)
    Baked Sweet Potato- 4 oz. (23gm carb)
    Butter or Margarine- 1 Tablespoon
    Banana Ice Cream- 2 serving (30gm carb)

24. *Breakfast 681 calories/60gm carb/54gm pro*
    French Toast - 2 serving (46gm carb)
    Berry Crush- 1 serving (8gm carb)
    Poached Egg- 1
    Greek Yogurt, plain – 6 oz. (6 gm carb)

Lunch 714 calories/61gm carb/42gm pro
Pork & Spanish Rice – 2 servings (42gm carb)
Refried Beans- 1/3 cup (10gm carb)
Raw Veggie Plate – 1 serving
Ranch Dressing - 2oz. (9gm carb)
Dinner 786 calories/60gm carb/49gm pro
Turkey Meatsauce -2 serving (12gm carb)
Whole Wheat Spaghetti- ¾ cup (28gm carb)
Caesar Salad – 1 serving (5gm carb)
Whole wheat Breadstick or Roll-1 (15gm carb)

25. *Breakfast 464 calories/62.5gm carb/24 gm pro*
Whole Wheat Cooked Cereal- 2/3 cup (22gm carb)
Whole Milk Plain Greek yogurt- 8 oz. (8 gm carb)
Ground Flaxseed- 1 Tablespoon (2.5 gm carb)
Butter or Margarine- 1 teaspoon
Banana- 1 large (30gm carb)
Lunch   727 calories/61.5gm carb/25gm pro
Pattie Melt w/caramelized onions- 1 serving (14 gm carb)
Ketchup- 1 Tablespoon (4gm carb)
Chopped Watermelon, diced- 1 cup (11.5gm carb)
Sweet potato chips- 2 oz. (32gm carb)
Dinner 589 calories/59 gm carb/34gm carb
Rotisserie Chicken
Roasted Asparagus
Baked Sweet Potato-5 oz. (29gm carb)
Butter or margarine- 1 Tablespoon
Chocolate Berries- 2 servings (30gm carb)

26. *Breakfast 412 calories/58gm carb/19gm pro*
Cheesy Eggs -1 serving
Mixed Grain Toast-3 slices (33gm carb)
Peach- 1 medium (16 gm carb)
Low sugar jelly- 1 Tablespoon (9gm carb)
Lunch 702 calories/44 gm carb/36gm pro
Taco Salad – 1 serving (26gm carb)
Sour Cream- ¼ cup (2gm carb)
Nectarine, large- 2 (32gm carb)

Dinner 662 calories/60gm carb/36gm pro
Pineapple Grilled Chicken- 1 serving (6.5gm carb)
Roasted Green Beans with Onions- 1 serving (2gm carb)
Wild rice, cooked- 2/3 cup (23gm carb)
Butter or margarine- 1 Tablespoon
Dark Chocolate- 8 pieces-24gm (28.5gm carb)

27. *Breakfast 492 calories/60gm carb/19gm pro*
    Veggie Omelet
    English Muffin- Whole Wheat -1.5 (40gm carb)
    Butter or Margarine- 1 Tablespoon
    Honeydew Melon. Diced- 1 cup (15gm carb)
    Low Sugar Jelly- 2 teaspoons (5gm carb)
    Lunch 655 calories/59gm carb/42gm pro
    Turkey Swiss Wrap – 1 serving (28 gm carb)
    Peach, medium-1 (14gm carb)
    Vegetable Chips- 1 oz. (17gm carb)
    Dinner 1005 calories/58gm/54gm pro
    Grilled Steak- 3 oz.
    Balsamic Mushrooms - 1 serving
    Tossed Salad- medium sized
    Salad Dressing- 1 oz. (5gm carb)
    Potato Skins – 2 servings (24gm carb)
    Wheat roll, small-1 (15gm carb)
    Watermelon, 1 ¼ cup diced (14gm carb)

28. *Breakfast 457 calories/60.5gm carb/22gm pro*
    Oat Bowl- 2 servings (29gm carb)
    Raisins- 2 Tablespoons (14.5gm carb)
    Canadian Bacon, grilled- 2 slices
    Wheat Toast- 1 slice (17gm carb)
    Butter or Margarine- 1 teaspoon
    Lunch 532 calories/61gm carb/18gm pro
    Hummus Lunch Bowl- (32gm Carb)
    Pita Bread-1 small (15gm carb)
    Blueberries- 2/3 cup (14gm carb)

__Dinner 644 calories/58gm carb/51gm pro__
Beef Chuck Roast- 5 oz.
Carrots, cooked with roast- ½ cup
Lima Beans- ½ cup (17.5gm carb)
Butter or margarine- 1 Tablespoon
Small Batch Cornbread – 2 serving (26gm carb)
Baked Pear- 1 serving (14.5 gm carb)

EASY RECIPES

SALADS

CAESAR SALAD
1 head romaine lettuce, cleaned and chopped
4 oz. sliced olives
4 oz. grated parmesan cheese
4 oz. croutons
Caesar dressing- ½ cup

Toss all ingredients in a medium bowl. Serves 6.
Per Serving
Calories: 234
Carbs: 8gm
Protein: 9gm
Fat: 19gm

CARIBBEAN COLESLAW
1 small package angel hair slaw mix (about 4 cups)
2-3 green onions, diced
3 Tablespoons cilantro, diced (optional)
2 Tablespoons light sour cream
2 Tablespoons light mayonnaise or salad dressing
2 Tablespoons lime juice
Hot sauce- optional

Combine slaw mix, onions (and cilantro, if desired) in a medium bowl.
Season with salt and pepper if desired and toss.
In a small bowl, combine sour cream, mayo, lime juice and hot sauce (if desired).
Toss together slaw and sour cream mixture.
Keep covered in refrigerator until ready to use.
Note: If you prefer a non-mayo based dressing, try dressing the slaw with rice wine vinegar sprinkled on top and a few drops of sesame oil. Mix the slaw and add more dressing as desired. (This will add no extra carbs.) Serves 4.
Per Serving
Calories: 52
Carbs: 1 gm
Protein: 1gm
Fat: 3 gm

COBB SALAD PLATTER
1 Head Romaine Lettuce, cleaned & chopped
6 slices bacon, cooked and chopped
4 large eggs, hardboiled, chopped
1 cup diced raw diced tomatoes
1 boneless chicken breast, roasted, chopped
1 avocado, peeled, pitted, chopped

Place lettuce on a large platter. Arrange remaining ingredients in rows on top of lettuce. Feel free to add rows of other low carb veggies such as radishes, green onions, celery, carrots, etc. Serves 4.
Per Serving:
Calories: 486
Carbs: 12gm
Protein: 55gm
Fat: 24gm

COLESLAW
½ cup coleslaw dressing
8 cups chopped cabbage
½ cup chopped green onion (optional)

Mix all ingredients in a large bowl. Store in refrigerator. Serves 8.
Per 3 oz. Serving:
Calories: 79 calories
Carbs: 8gm
Protein: 1gm
Fat: 5gm

EASY GREEK CHICKEN SALAD BOWL
4 <u>Easy Greek Chicken Breasts</u>, cooked and sliced
8 cups fresh spinach
2 cups diced tomatoes
6 oz. sliced olives
1 cup crumbled feta cheese

Divide all ingredients between 4 large salad bowls. Serves 4.
Per Serving:
Calories: 349
Carbs: (carbs are from free foods)
Protein: 34 gm
Fat: 19gm

GREEK CHICKEN CHOPPED SALAD

4 <u>Easy Greek Chicken Breasts</u>, cooked and chopped coarsely
1 head romaine, chopped
3 celery ribs, chopped
1 medium cucumber, chopped
½ cup grated parmesan cheese
½ cup oil & vinegar dressing
½ cup wheat croutons

Combine all ingredients in a large salad bowl and toss lightly to combine. Serves 4.
Per Serving:
Calories: 391
Carbs: 11 gm
Protein: 32gm
Fat:25gm

SPINACH SALAD

4 cups fresh spinach
½ cup mushrooms, sliced
¼ cup red onion, Sliced
¼ cup Walnuts, chopped
¼ cup oil & vinegar or raspberry vinaigrette dressing
Grilled Chicken or Grilled Shrimp (optional)

Combine all ingredients in a large salad bowl and toss lightly. Serves 4.
Per Serving:
Calories: 134
Carbs: (carbs are from free foods)
Protein: 6gm
Fat: 11gm

SUMMER CORN SALAD
    1 can whole kernel corn, drained
    1 small box cherry tomatoes, halved
    1 medium cucumber, peeled and chopped
    6 green onions, chopped
    3 Tablespoons mayonnaise

Combine all ingredients and season to taste with salt, pepper or your favorite all-purpose seasoning. Refrigerate for several hours for best flavor. Serves 4.
Per Serving:
Calories: 120
Carbs: 19gm
Protein: 3gm
Fat: 5gm

TACO SALAD
    1# Lean Ground Beef (93% lean)
    1 package (1.25oz.) taco seasoning mix, dry
    3 oz. Tortilla Chips
    2 cups shredded lettuce
    2 cups diced Tomatoes
    1 cup grated cheddar cheese, Mexican blend
    ½ cup Salsa

Cook ground beef and add taco seasoning per directions on package. Divide chips between 4 large salad bowls. Divide taco meat between salads and layer over chips. Next add layers of lettuce, tomato, cheese and salsa, dividing evenly among bowls. Garnish with a spoonful of sour cream if desired. Serve immediately. Serves 4.
Per Serving:
Calories: 454
Carbs: 26gm
Protein: 31gm
Fat: 24gm

SANDWICHES AND WRAPS

APPLE NUT SANDWICH
1 small apple, sliced
Lemon Juice, optional
2 Tablespoons peanut butter
1 Tablespoon Coconut
1 Tablespoon chocolate chips or raisins

Slice apple into four pieces. Brush each apple slice lightly with lemon juice, if desired, to prevent browning. Place 2 slices of apple onto a plate and spread 1 Tablespoon peanut butter evenly onto each slice. Sprinkle coconut and chocolate chips over the peanut butter and top with remaining 2 slices apple. Serves 1.
Per Serving:
Calories: 297
Carbohydrates: 31gm
Protein: 9gm
Fat: 18gm

CHEESE TOAST
1 slice whole wheat thin bread (8gm carb/slice)
1 teaspoon butter or margarine
1 thin slice cheddar cheese

Spread butter on bread and toast lightly. Add cheese slice and melt. Serves 1.
Per Serving:
Calories: 178
Carbohydrates: 8gm
Protein: 9gm
Fat: 12gm

GREEK CHICKEN SALAD STUFFED PITA
1 recipe Greek Chicken Salad
2 lower carb pita breads (10 gm carb each), warmed
1 cup fresh spinach
½ cup sliced tomato

Divide chicken salad between pita breads and top with lettuce and tomato. Serves 2.
Per Serving:
Calories: 319
Carbs: 12gm
Protein: 16gm
Fat: 17gm

GREEK CHICKEN SANDWICH

1 recipe <u>Easy Greek Chicken</u>, cooked
4 lower carb sandwich rolls
½ cup prepared pesto
Small jar roasted red peppers
4 thin slices mozzarella cheese

Place a chicken breast on each roll and divide remaining ingredients among sandwiches. Place under broiler or in toaster oven just until cheese melts and sandwich is thoroughly warmed. Serves 4.
Per Serving:
Calories: 419
Carbs: 22gm
Protein: 43gm
Fat: 16gm

GREEK CHICKEN WRAP

4 low-carb pita wraps, warmed
1 recipe <u>Easy Greek Chicken</u>, cooked and sliced
2 cups shredded lettuce
1 cup diced tomatoes
2 Tablespoons Caesar or Italian dressing
4 Tablespoons olives (optional)

Place a pita bread on each of four plates. Divide all ingredients evenly between pitas and serve warm. Serves 4.
Per Serving:
Calories: 300
Carbs: 13gm
Protein: 33gm
Fat: 14gm

GRILLED SHRIMP WRAP

1 small tortilla
3 oz. grilled shrimp
½ cup shredded lettuce
½ cup diced tomatoes
2 Tablespoons ranch dressing

Heat tortilla or lower carb wrap per label directions. Add remaining items to tortilla and roll up to contain filling. Serves 1
Per Serving:
Calories: 319
Carbs: 28gm
Protein: 26gm
Fat: 12gm

TURKEY SWISS WRAP

1 multigrain tortilla, warmed
3 oz. Sliced turkey
1 slice Swiss Cheese
½ cup Lettuce & 1/3 cup Tomato
2 Tablespoons Ranch Dressing

Place tortilla on a flat surface and layer ingredients as listed. Roll up tortilla and secure with toothpick if desired. Serves 1.
Per Serving:
Calories: 462
Carbs: 25gm
Protein: 39gm
Fat: 21gm

EGGS AND BREAKFAST DISHES

BREAKFAST BANANA SPLIT

¼ banana (3 oz.), sliced lengthwise
6 oz. Greek yogurt, plain, nonfat
1 Tablespoon chopped nuts
2 Tablespoons whipped cream, sugar free
1 strawberry

In a small bowl, place sliced banana and layer remaining ingredients in order listed. Serves 1.

Per Serving
Calories: 282
Carbohydrates: 31gm
Protein: 21gm
Fat: 10gm

BREAKFAST BURRITO

1 flour tortilla
1 Recipe Easy Eggs
2 Tablespoon diced green pepper
2 oz. turkey sausage, cooked and crumbled
½ cup cheddar or pepper-jack cheese

Heat tortilla according to label instructions. Stuff tortilla with remaining ingredients and fold up burrito style. Serves 1.
Per Serving
Calories: 398
Carbs: 17gm
Protein: 29gm
Fat: 23gm

CHEESY EGGS

1 Recipe Easy Eggs
¼ cup grated cheese

Follow recipe for Easy Eggs adding cheese while cooking. Serves 2.
Per Serving:
Calories: 103
Carbs: 1gm
Protein: 7gm
Fat: 8gm

CINNAMON TOAST

2 slices wheat bread, diet (8-10gm carb/slice)
1 Tablespoon butter or margarine
½ teaspoon ground cinnamon

Toast bread and spread with butter. Sprinkle with cinnamon as desired.
Serves 1
Per Serving:
Calories: 172
Carbs: 20gm
Protein: 7gm
Fat: 9gm

COUNTRY EGG SANDWICH

2 eggs
4 slices thin bread (8-10gm carb/slice)
2 teaspoons butter or margarine
1 small tomato, sliced thinly (optional)
salt & pepper, as desired

Heat eggs in a non-stick skillet over medium heat until cooked. Spread margarine on toast and brown under broiler. Place an egg between 2 slices toast and serve with tomatoes (as desired). Serves 2

Per Serving:
Calories: 195
Carbs: 20gm
Protein: 13gm
Fat: 9gm

DEVILED EGGS

3 eggs, boiled and peeled
1 Tablespoon mayo
1 Tablespoon pickle relish
1 teaspoon prepared mustard
1/8 teaspoon salt
Paprika (optional)

Cut eggs in half and scoop out yolk into small bowl. Mash yolk with a fork and add remaining ingredients and stir to combine. Adjust seasoning by adding salt & pepper as desired. Spoon mixture back into egg white halves and garnish with paprika if desired. Serves 3.
Per Serving:
Calories: 103cal
Carbs: 2 gm
Protein: 6 gm
Fat: 7 gm

EASY EGGS

2 eggs
1 Tablespoon milk or cream
Salt and pepper as desired
1 teaspoon butter or oil

Combine first 3 ingredients and beat lightly with a fork until well combined. Heat butter over low to medium heat in non-stick pan until melted. Add eggs and cook, stirring occasionally, until set. Serves 2
Per Serving:
Calories: 93
Carbs: 1gm
Protein: 7gm
Fat: 7gm

EGG BAKED IN AVOCADO CUPS
　　1 Avocado
　　2 eggs
　　Salt and pepper

Preheat oven to 425 degrees F. Cut avocados in half, then scoop out space in each half to hold egg (about 2 Tablespoons). Place avocados in a small baking pan. Sprinkle avocado with salt and pepper as desired. Carefully break egg into each avocado half.
Bake until egg is set- about 12-16 minutes. Optional: Sprinkle egg with bacon bits, chives, or cheese if desired. Serves 2.
Per Serving:
Calories: 232
Carbs: 9gm
Protein: 8gm
Fat: 19gm

EGGS BENEDICT
　　4 English Muffin halves
　　1 Tbsp. Butter or Margarine
　　4 eggs, cooked over easy or poached (avoid undercooked yolks)
　　4 slices lean ham
　　1 pkg. hollandaise sauce, prepared per label directions

Spread butter on muffin halves and toast. Top with ham slice then egg. Drizzle with 2 Tablespoons sauce. Serves 4.
Per Serving:
Calories: 241
Carbs: 17gm
Protein: 16gm
Fat: 12gm

EGGS IN HAM CUPS
　　6 slices ham
　　6 eggs
　　Grated cheese (optional)

Preheat oven to 375 degrees F. Spray a muffin tin with non-stick spray and line each cup with a slice of ham. Crack egg into each ham cup and sprinkle with salt and pepper as desired. (Optional- top with grated cheese if desired.) Bake until egg is set- approximately 15-20 minutes. Serves 6.

Per Serving:
Calories: 115
Carbs: 0
Protein: 12gm
Fat: 7gm

ENGLISH MUFFIN STACK

1 English Muffin, toasted with butter (if desired)
1 Egg in Ham Cup

Place one English muffin half on a plate and top with egg in ham cup and remaining toasted English muffin half on top to form sandwich. Serves 1.
Per Serving:
Calories: 311
Carbs: 26gm
Protein: 18gm
Fat: 15gm

FRENCH TOAST

4 slices thin bread (7-10gm carb/slice)
2 eggs, beaten
Dash salt
1 teaspoon vanilla
½ cup milk
1/8 teaspoon ground cinnamon
Butter or margarine (optional)

Combine all ingredients (except bread) in an 8-9" square pan. Stir to combine. Lay bread in pan and flip to coat both sides well. Allow bread to soak 10-20 minutes (or overnight) until all egg mixture is absorbed. Place bread on a parchment coated baking pan and sprinkle with extra cinnamon and a pat of butter, as desired. Cook at 350 degrees F approximately 15-20 minutes or until lightly browned. (May flip toast halfway through baking for even cooking.) Serves 2.
Per Serving:
Calories: 204
Carbs: 23gm
Protein: 14gm
Fat: 7gm

GREEK YOGURT PARFAIT

4 oz. Greek Yogurt
¼ cup blueberries (fresh or frozen)
½ teaspoon ground flaxseed
1/3 cup granola (20gm carb/serving or less)

In a small bowl, layer ingredients in order listed. Serve immediately or cover and chill for use later. Serves 1
Per Serving:
Calories: 227
Carbs: 32gm
Protein: 12gm
Fat: 7gm

HAM, EGG AND VEGGIE ROLL UP

1 teaspoon olive oil
2 Mushrooms, cleaned and thinly sliced
¼ cup diced green peppers
1 stalk green onion, chopped
1 Egg, slightly beaten
1 oz. diced turkey ham
Salsa (optional)

Heat olive oil in a small non-stick pan over medium heat, add veggies and cook until tender 3-5 minutes.
Remove veggies from pan and add oil as needed to lightly coat pan. Pour egg in pan. Allow egg to set without stirring, 3-5 minutes. Top with cooked veggies and ham. Roll up egg to contain filling and serve. Serves 1.
Per Serving:
Calories: 165
Carbs: (carbs are from free foods)
Protein: 13gm
Fat: 11gm

HIGH PROTEIN OATMEAL

½ cup quick-cooking oatmeal (uncooked)
½ teaspoon salt (optional)
1 Tablespoon ground flaxseed
1 cup almond milk, unsweetened
1 egg, slightly beaten
Cinnamon (optional)

Combine oatmeal, salt, and flaxseed in a small sauce pan. Add milk and egg to pan and stir well. Bring to a simmer, stirring occasionally, and cook 2-3 minutes or until mixture reaches 160 degrees F (to fully cook egg). Sprinkle with cinnamon if desired and serve. Serves 2.
Per Serving:
Calories: 140
Carbs: 15gm
Protein: 7gm
Fat: 6gm

OAT BOWL

½ cup cooked oatmeal
1 teaspoon butter
¼- ½ teaspoon cinnamon (optional)
2 teaspoons sliced almonds

Pour cooked oatmeal into bowl and add butter and cinnamon. Stir well and sprinkle with almonds. Serves 1.
Per Serving:
Calories: 100
Carbs: 15gm
Protein: 3gm
Fat: 4gm

OATMEAL BANANA SMOOTHIE

½ cup oatmeal, uncooked
1 cup almond milk
6 oz. Greek yogurt, plain
½ teaspoon cinnamon
1 medium banana, sliced and frozen
6 medium strawberries, frozen

Combine all ingredients in a blender and pulse until smooth. Serves 3.
Per Serving:
Calories: 157
Carbs: 28gm
Protein: 9gm
Fat: 2gm

SWEET POTATO BREAKFAST CUPS

19 oz. package frozen sweet potato tots
Oil for greasing muffin tin
½ cup lean diced turkey ham
4 eggs
1 Tablespoon milk

Preheat oven to 400 degrees F. Line a 6 muffin tin with muffin liners- coat liners with non-stick spray. Allow tots to thaw (or thaw in microwave) then place about 5-6 tots in each cup. Mash tots with back of spoon or small glass to form cup shape in muffin tin. Bake for 10 minutes. (Monitor baking to avoid over-browning) Remove cups from oven and lower oven temperature to 350 degrees. Add diced ham to cups, dividing evenly. Mix eggs and milk until evenly combined, add salt and pepper as desired. Divide egg mixture between muffin cups. Bake cups for 10-15 minutes or until eggs are set. Serves 6.
Per Serving:
Calories: 210
Carbs: 28gm
Protein: 8gm
Fat: 7gm

VEGGIE OMELET

2 eggs
1 Tablespoon light cream or whole milk
1 teaspoon olive oil or butter (divided)
½ cup diced veggies (peppers, onions, mushrooms, etc.)
2 Tablespoons grated cheddar cheese

Combine first 2 ingredients and add salt and pepper as desired. Beat slightly. Add 1 teaspoon olive oil to a non-stick skillet and heat over medium until warm add veggies and sauté until tender. Remove from skillet and set aside. Add a small amount of oil to skillet to coat lightly. Add eggs to skillet and cook on low-medium heat until eggs are set. Sprinkle sautéed veggies on top of one half of eggs and top with cheese. Fold other half of eggs over veggie/cheese to form omelet. Heat until cheese melts. Serves 2.
Per Serving:

Calories: 137
Carbs: (carbs are from free foods)
Protein: 9gm
Fat: 10gm

MAIN DISHES

BALSAMIC PORK TENDERLOIN

1# pork tenderloin
2 Tablespoons balsamic vinegar
1 Tablespoon Dijon mustard
1 teaspoon thyme
Salt & Pepper, as desired

Trim tenderloin and place in re-sealable plastic bag along with remaining ingredients. Allow to marinate 20-30 minutes, then place tenderloin on a foil-lined rimmed baking sheet. Preheat oven to 475 degrees F. Roast approximately 20 minutes or until internal temperature registers 145 degrees on meat thermometer. To prevent over-browning, may cover loosely with foil. Serves 4.

Per Serving:
Calories: 134
Carbs: 2gm
Protein: 24gm
Fat: 3gm

CHICKEN (OR PORK) & VEGGIE STIR FRY

1 Tablespoon corn starch
½ cup cold or room temp lower sodium chicken broth
2 Tablespoons low sodium soy sauce
1 Tablespoon + 1 teaspoon olive oil, divided
1# Chicken Breast, raw, diced or 1# pork tenderloin, raw, sliced thin
16 oz. Chinese vegetables, frozen
1/8 teaspoon ground ginger (optional)

Place cornstarch in a small bowl. Add about 2-3 Tablespoons of the chicken broth and stir until cornstarch is dissolved. Add the rest of chicken broth and the soy sauce. Stir well and set aside.

Heat 1 tablespoon olive oil in a non-stick skillet over medium heat and add chicken and stir fry until fully cooked. Remove from skillet. Add remaining 1 teaspoon olive oil to skillet and add veggies and ginger. Stir fry veggies until tender- 3-5 minutes. Stir broth mixture and add to skillet. Cook and stir veggie and broth mixture 2-3 minutes and allow to simmer and thicken slightly. Add chicken back to skillet and stir to combine. Serves 4.

Per Serving:
Calories: 314
Carbs: (carbs are from free foods)
Protein: 28gm
Fat: 8gm

CRUNCHY FISH TACOS WITH CARIBBEAN SLAW

1 recipe Easy Baked Fish
1 recipe Caribbean Coleslaw
4 Corn Tortillas (warmed)

Divide fish fillets between tortillas and top with coleslaw. Serve with lime wedges. Serves 2.
Per Serving
Calories: 268
Carbs: 32gm
Protein: 17gm
Fat: 9gm

EASY BAKED FISH

2 medium fish fillets
Lower sodium Old Bay seasoning
Paprika
Salt and pepper, as desired

Preheat oven to 375 degrees F. Place fish fillets on a foil lined baking pan. Sprinkle fish with seasonings on both sides and cook until fork tender approximately 20-25 minutes. Serves 2
Per Serving:
Calories: 102
Carbs: 0
Protein: 13gm
Fat: 5gm

EASY GREEK CHICKEN
4 chicken breasts, raw, approximately 4 oz. each*
1 Tablespoon olive oil
1 Tablespoon balsamic vinegar
½ teaspoon oregano
½ teaspoon minced garlic
¼ teaspoon thyme
Salt and pepper

Salt and pepper (if desired) chicken breasts, then combine with remaining ingredients in a large freezer bag. Allow to marinate up to 24 hours. Place chicken in a sauté pan coated with non-stick spray and heated to medium. Cook chicken, turning occasionally until all sides are golden brown and temperature reads 165 degrees (approx. 7-10 min depending upon thickness). Store in refrigerator up to 3 days or freeze. Serves 4. *Chicken breasts will have best flavor if each breast is sliced crosswise into 2-3 thin slices before marinating.
Per Serving:
Calories: 171
Carbs: 1gm
Protein: 26 gm
Fat: 6gm

EGGPLANT PARM
1 small eggplant
½ cup panko breadcrumbs
½ cup grated parmesan cheese
1 egg, slightly beaten with 2 Tbsp. water
1 recipe Easy Marinara Sauce or 3 cups lower carb bottled spaghetti sauce
1 cup mozzarella cheese, divided

Preheat oven to 375 degrees F. Line a large cookie sheet with parchment paper or spray with non-stick spray. Peel eggplant and slice into ¼- ½ " rounds. Mix panko and cheese in a shallow bowl and place egg in another small, shallow bowl. Dip eggplant into egg and allow excess to drip off, then roll in crumb mixture. Place each coated eggplant slice on baking sheet. Bake for 20-30 minutes until browned and tender. (May turn slices over halfway through baking for even browning.) In 8" or 9" baking dish, pour about 1 cup marinara. Lay eggplant slices over sauce, then sprinkle with ¾ cup mozzarella cheese. Cover with remaining marinara then sprinkle remaining mozzarella cheese on top. Bake for 20 minutes or until hot and bubbly. Serves 6

Per Serving:
Calories: 148
Carbs: 16gm
Protein: 11gm
Fat: 8gm

FAVORITE TACOS

1# lean ground beef
1 pkg. taco seasoning
6 corn tortilla shells
Veggies (lettuce, tomato, onions)
1 cup shredded cheese
Salsa (optional)

Prepare ground beef with taco seasoning per package directions. Meanwhile, warm tortilla shells as directed on label. Serve with veggies, cheese and salsa as desired. Serves 3 (2 tacos per serving)
Per Serving:
Calories: 506
Carbs: 33gm
Protein: 41gm
Fat: 25gm

FLATBREAD PIZZA

1 focaccia Italian flatbread, plain (about 20 carbs or less/flatbread)
1 teaspoon olive oil
¼ cup pizza sauce
½ -1 cup chopped veggies (peppers, onions, mushrooms, etc.)
¼ cup sliced olives
½ cup mozzarella cheese

Preheat oven as directed on flatbread label. Spread pizza sauce on flatbread and add remaining ingredients. Cook per label recommendations or until bread is crispy and cheese is melted. Serves 1.
Per Serving:
Calories: 419
Carbs: 28gm
Protein: 21gm
Fat: 24gm

FRIED RICE
2 teaspoons oil
1 cup diced veggies (celery, onions, mushrooms, etc.)
1/3 cup cooked and chilled brown rice
½ cup diced leftover meat
Soy Sauce, to taste

In a medium size non-stick skillet, heat oil over medium-high heat. Add veggies and stir fry until crisp tender. Add remaining ingredients and stir fry 3-4 minutes or until well heated. Serves 1.
Per Serving:
Calories: 428
Carbs: 24gm
Protein: 35gm
Fat: 21gm

GREEK CHICKEN SALAD
1 cup diced Easy Greek Chicken
2 Tablespoons mayonnaise or Greek yogurt
¼ cup crumbled feta cheese
2 Tablespoons chopped olives
Salt and pepper, as desired

Combine all ingredients in a medium bowl and stir to combine. Adjust seasonings and add extra mayo if desired. Serves 2
Per Serving:
Calories: 271
Carbs: 2 gm
Protein: 27gm
Fat: 17gm

GRILLED BBQ PORK CHOP
4 pork chops (about 1# total), bone in, trimmed of excess fat (at least ¾"thick)
BBQ Dry Rub Seasoning (or your favorite brand, 0 carb)
Oil for coating grill if needed

Sprinkle chops liberally with rub and place in plastic bag. Seal bag and place in refrigerator for up to 4 hours to marinate. About 15-20 minutes before placing on grill, remove chops from refrigerator and place on counter. Prepare grill and bring to medium heat . Cook chops until meat thermometer reads 145 degrees- approximately 15-20 minutes.   Serves 4.

Per Serving:
Calories: 189
Carbs: 1gm
Protein: 25gm
Fat: 9gm

HERB ROASTED CHICKEN & VEGGIES

1 chicken
3-4 carrots, cut into 2-3" pieces
8-10 fresh mushrooms
2-3 ribs celery, cut into 2-3" pieces
Herb seasoning

Preheat oven to 375 degrees F. Place chicken in a foil lined baking dish and sprinkle with salt and pepper as desired. Add veggies to pan. Sprinkle chicken with herb seasoning and roast 45-50 minutes or until meat thermometer registers 165 degrees in thigh meat. May cover lightly with foil if needed to prevent over-browning. Allow to set for 5-10 minutes before serving. Serves 6.

Per Serving
Calories: 228
Carbs: (carbs are from free foods)
Protein: 40gm
Fat: 6gm

HUMMUS LUNCH BOWL

½ cup prepared hummus
1 teaspoon olive oil
¼ cup sliced olives
1/3 cup diced tomatoes
Carrot and celery sticks
1 small whole grain pita (about 15 carbs/pita), cut into wedges

Place hummus in bowl and drizzle with olive oil. Top with olives and tomatoes. Serve with veggie sticks and warm pita wedges for dipping. Serves 1.

Per Serving:
Calories: 328
Carbs: 32gm
Protein: 14gm
Fat: 21gm

JERK CHICKEN

½ chicken, raw
½ -1 Tablespoon Jerk Seasoning

Preheat oven to 375 degrees F. Coat chicken with seasoning and place in a foil-lined baking pan. Roast chicken for 45 minutes to 1 hour or until thermometer placed in thickest part of chicken registers 165 degrees. Serves 2.
Per Serving:
Calories: 196
Carbs: 0
Protein: 35gm
Fat: 5gm

LIGHTER LASAGNA CAPRESE

4 lasagna noodles- preferably whole grain, cooked
1 recipe Easy Marinara Sauce (divided)
8 oz. ricotta cheese
3-4 Roma tomatoes, sliced thinly
4 oz. mozzarella cheese block, or sliced mozzarella cheese
8-10 fresh basil leaves

Preheat oven to 350 degrees F. Slice cooked noodles in half. Mix 1 cup marinara sauce with ½ cup ricotta cheese. Spread 2 Tablespoons ricotta/sauce mixture onto each noodle half. Top with 3 tomato slices. Top tomato slices with a teaspoon size piece of mozzarella then sprinkle a torn basil leaf over mozzarella. Roll up noodle and place in a 9" pie pan. Repeat process with remaining 7 noodle halves. Pour about 1 cup remaining marinara sauce over all (to cover pasta and prevent over-browning) then top with grated mozzarella cheese. Bake uncovered for about 30 minutes or until sauce is bubbly. Serves 4.
Per Serving:
Calories: 316
Carbs: 28gm
Protein: 19gm
Fat: 16gm

OPEN FACED LOADED BURGERS
½ # ground beef, lean
1 tsp. Worcestershire sauce
Olive oil
1 cup raw veggies (mushrooms, onions, peppers)
2 thin slices cheese
1 hamburger bun, preferably whole grain

Form beef into 2 patties and season with Worcestershire sauce and black pepper (as desired). Heat a non-stick skillet medium and add beef patties. Cook until internal temperature reads 160 degrees F on meat thermometer. Remove patties from skillet and add enough olive oil to lightly coat skillet then add veggies. Cook veggies until crisp tender. Toast bun halves. Top each bun half with a beef pattie, 1/2 of veggies then cheese slice. Place under broiler to melt cheese.
Serves 2.
Per Serving:
Calories: 452
Carbs: 14gm
Protein: 31gm
Fat: 30gm

OVEN BAKED BBQ RIBS
2# country-style ribs (trimmed of fat)
½ -1 Tablespoon BBQ rub seasoning

Preheat oven to 350 degrees F. Sprinkle ribs with BBQ rub seasoning. Place ribs in a foil-lined pan and cover with foil. Bake for 1 1/4- 1 1/2 hours or until very tender. Remove foil and broil for 4-6 minutes to add crispy crust if desired.
Serves 6.
Per Serving:
Calories: 215
Carbs: 1gm
Protein: 32gm
Fat: 9gm

PATTY MELT WITH CARAMELIZED ONIONS
½# lean ground beef
1 teaspoon Worcestershire Sauce
1 small onion, sliced
1 whole grain hamburger bun, toasted or steamed

Divide beef into 2 patties and season with Worcestershire sauce and ground black pepper (as desired). Place beef patties and sliced onion in a non-stick skillet and cook over medium heat until meat thermometer placed in thickest part of a beef patty registers 160 degrees F and onions are brown and tender. To serve: place ½ hamburger bun on plate and top with a patty and onions. Serves 2.
Per Serving:
Calories: 363
Carbs: 14gm
Protein: 22gm
Fat: 24gm

PINEAPPLE GRILLED CHICKEN
4 chicken breasts (approx. 4 oz. each)
2 oz. teriyaki sauce (lower sodium)
2 Tablespoons lemon juice
1 teaspoon minced garlic
4 slices pineapple

Combine all ingredients except pineapple in a large sealed freezer bag and marinate up to 8 hours in refrigerator. Preheat grill or non-stick skillet (add 1-2 tsp. oil to skillet) and add drained chicken breasts and pineapple slices. Cook until pineapple and chicken are browned slightly and chicken registers 165 degrees on a meat thermometer. Serves 4.
Per Serving:
Calories: 166
Carbs: 7gm
Protein: 27gm
Fat: 3gm

PORK & SPANISH RICE
½ Tablespoon Olive Oil
½ # pork tenderloin, raw, sliced ¼" thick
8 oz. lower sodium chicken broth
½ cup quick-cooking brown rice, uncooked
½ cup mild salsa
1/3 cup shredded cheddar cheese

Heat olive oil in non-stick skillet over medium heat. Season tenderloin with salt and pepper (if desired). Add pork to skillet and quickly brown both sides, remove from skillet and set aside. Add rice to skillet and add chicken broth and salsa. Stir well. Layer tenderloin on top of rice mixture and cover skillet. Cook rice and tenderloin as directed on rice label or until pork registers 145 degrees on thermometer and rice is tender. Fluff rice and serve with cheddar cheese sprinkled over all. Serves 4.
Per Serving:
Calories: 218
Carbs: 21gm
Protein: 17gm
Fat: 7gm

PORK TENDERLOIN WITH APPLES

½ teaspoon paprika
½ teaspoon rosemary, crushed
½ teaspoon garlic powder
¼ teaspoon salt
1 medium pork tenderloin (about 1 pound)
1 oz. apple juice, unsweetened
2 medium apples, cut into thin slices

Preheat oven to 425 degrees. Combine first 4 ingredients in a plastic bag. Moisten pork slightly with apple juice and place in bag with seasoning. Shake bag to coat pork then remove pork from bag and place in a medium size foil-lined baking pan. (Discard bag.) Arrange apple slices around pork and roast 20-25 minutes or until meat thermometer registers 145 degrees F. (May cover loosely with foil to prevent over-browning if needed.) Allow pork to rest on counter for 4-5 minutes before serving. Serves 5.
Per Serving:
Calories: 141
Carbs: 11gm
Protein: 19gm
Fat: 2gm

RED & WHITE CHICKEN CHILI

1 teaspoon olive oil
¼ cup diced onion (may use frozen)
½ cup mild chilies and tomatoes
1 Tablespoon cornstarch
1 teaspoon ground cumin
1 (16 oz.) can Northern beans (drained)
1 cup chicken broth
1 cup cooked diced chicken

In a medium saucepan, heat olive oil until warm and add onions. Cook onions until tender, about 3-4 minutes. Add chilies and tomatoes, cornstarch and cumin. Stir to combine then simmer for 2-3 minutes, stirring occasionally. Add beans, chicken broth, and chicken then bring to a simmer or low boil and cook 5-7 minutes or until thickened. Serves 6.
Per Serving:
Calories: 194
Carbs: 30gm
Protein: 17gm
Fat: 2gm

ROTISSERIE CHICKEN

2 chicken breasts, raw (4 oz. each)
Rotisserie Chicken Seasoning

Preheat oven to 375 degrees F. Line a small baking pan with foil. Sprinkle chicken with seasoning and bake until meat thermometer registers 165 degrees on a meat thermometer, approximately 20-30 minutes. Serves 2.
Per Serving:
Calories: 155
Carbs: 0
Protein: 26gm
Fat: 5gm

SALMON PATTIES

1 (7.5 oz.) can Alaskan salmon
1 egg
1 green onion, diced
¼ cup unbleached wheat flour
¾ teaspoon baking powder
½ -1 Tablespoon olive oil

Drain salmon, reserving 1 Tablespoon juice. Mix salmon, egg and onion. Stir in flour until well blended. Combine reserved salmon juice and baking powder and stir until bubbly. Add to salmon mixture and stir gently to combine. Shape into small patties (approx. 1/4 cup or 2.8 oz.). Heat olive oil in a medium sized non-stick pan and cook patties until lightly browned- about 4 minutes each side. (May add extra olive oil if needed.) Serves 4.
Per Serving:
Calories: 163
Carbs: 6gm
Protein: 15gm
Fat: 9gm

STEAK KABOBS

8 oz. sirloin steak, raw, cut into 2" cubes
1 small pkg. mushrooms caps, cleaned and stems removed
2 medium bell peppers, cut into 2" pieces
1 medium onion, cut into 2" pieces
1-2 Tablespoons Soy Sauce
1 clove garlic, minced

Place all ingredients (including salt & pepper as desired) in a zip top bag and allow to marinate in refrigerator 2-3 hours. Drain ingredients and thread onto four 10-12" metal skewers. Discard marinade. Grill until beef pieces are to desired doneness. Serves 3.
Per Serving:
Calories: 209
Carbs: (carbs are from free foods)
Protein: 20gm
Fat: 10gm

TORTILLA PIZZA
1 Low Carb Tortilla
2 Tablespoons Pizza Sauce
½ cup chopped Veggies (peppers, onions, mushrooms, etc.)
1 Tablespoon sliced olives
1/3 cup mozzarella cheese

Preheat oven to 350 degrees F. Place tortilla on baking sheet and heat 3-4 minutes. Tortilla will be slightly crispy- watch tortilla closely to prevent over-browning. Remove tortilla from oven and add toppings in order listed. Return to oven and bake 5-6 minutes or until cheese is melted. Serves 1.
Per Serving:
Calories: 246
Carbs: 24gm
Protein: 13gm
Fat: 11gm

TURKEY DIVAN
1 10 oz. package frozen broccoli
2 Tablespoons butter
2 Tablespoons unbleached flour
½ teaspoon chicken bouillon granules
1 cup milk
4-6 slices fully cooked, sliced turkey breast (about ¼ " thick) or leftover chicken breast, sliced
¼ cup grated parmesan cheese (optional)

Preheat oven to 375 degrees F. Cook broccoli per directions on label then allow to drain. (If you prefer firm broccoli, undercook slightly as broccoli will cook further in oven.) In a small saucepan, melt butter and whisk in flour and bouillon. Allow to cook at a low simmer a few minutes then slowly whisk in milk. Return to a simmer or low boil. Cook 2-3 minutes, stirring occasionally. Taste sauce and adjust seasoning with salt and pepper as needed.
Spread drained broccoli out in 8" or 9" metal pan. Pour ½ sauce over broccoli then layer turkey slices over. Pour remaining sauce over turkey. Sprinkle with cheese if desired. Place in preheated oven to cook about 15-20 minutes or until bubbly. Turn oven to broil and allow cheese to brown if desired. Serves 4.

Per Serving:
Calories: 282
Carbs: 10gm
Protein: 41gm
Fat: 9gm

TURKEY MEATSAUCE

1 teaspoon olive oil
1# lean ground turkey
1 recipe Easy Marinara Sauce

Add olive oil to a non-stick skillet and heat. Add ground turkey and stir over medium heat until browned and thoroughly cooked. Add Easy Marinara Sauce and stir to combine with turkey. Serves 6.
Per Serving:
Calories: 152
Carbs: 6gm
Protein: 15gm
Fat: 8gm

VERACRUZ STYLE SNAPPER

1 teaspoon olive oil
¼ cup chopped onion
1 clove garlic, minced
2/3 cup cherry tomatoes
¼ cup sliced green olives
1 teaspoon dried oregano leaves
6 oz. Red Snapper or other white fish fillet
1 oz. lime juice (optional)

Preheat oven to 400 degrees F. Heat olive oil over medium heat in a non-stick skillet. Add onions and garlic and cook until onions become slightly tender, about 5-6 minutes. Add remaining ingredients (except fish and lime juice) and cook until tomatoes soften, about 4-5 minutes. Spray a small baking dish with non-stick spray. Cut snapper filet in half and sprinkle with salt & pepper if desired. Place fillets in baking dish and top with tomato mixture. Sprinkle with lime juice (if desired) and cook until fish is tender and flakes easily- about 20 minutes depending upon thickness. Serves 2.

Per Serving:
Calories: 149
Carbs: 7gm
Protein: 18gm
Fat: 5gm

VEGETABLES AND SIDE DISHES

BALSAMIC MUSHROOMS

1 teaspoon olive oil
1 cup sliced mushrooms
1 Tablespoon balsamic vinegar

In medium non-stick skillet, heat olive oil and add sliced mushrooms. Stir and cook 4-5 minutes then add balsamic vinegar. Stir and cook another 1-2 minutes until tender. Serves 1.
Per Serving:
Calories: 69
Carbs: (carbs are from free foods)
Protein: 2gm
Fat: 5gm

BROCCOLI TOSS

1 ½ Tablespoons olive oil
1 Tablespoon lemon juice
¼ cup parmesan cheese
Salt & Pepper to taste
3 cups steamed or roasted broccoli

Combine first 4 ingredients and mix well. Pour over hot broccoli and toss to coat. Serves 6.
Per Serving:
Calories: 72
Carbs: (carbs are from free foods)
Protein: 3gm
Fat: 5gm

POTATO SKINS

4 medium-size potatoes, baked
2 teaspoons butter or margarine or olive oil
2 teaspoons chopped bacon
½ cup shredded cheese
Salt & Pepper as desired
Sour Cream (optional)

Preheat oven to 350 degrees F. Scoop out potatoes (reserve potato for another meal) leaving skins. Place skins on a foil lined baking sheet. Brush with butter or olive oil and lightly season with salt and pepper. Bake skins 8-10 minutes. Remove skins and sprinkle with bacon and cheese. Place under broiler until cheese is melted. Serve with sour cream and diced green onions, if desired. Serves 2.
Per Serving:
Calories: 233
Carbs: 12gm
Protein: 12gm
Fat: 15gm

RAW VEGGIE PLATE
3 medium baby carrots
¼ cup sliced radish
3 medium celery stalks, cut into sticks
½ cup raw cauliflower- chopped into bite-size pieces

Wash and drain veggies. Arrange on a small platter. Serves 1.
Per Serving:
Calories: 36
Carbs: (carbs are from free foods)
Protein: 2gm
Fat: 0

ROASTED CHERRY TOMATOES
1 box cherry tomatoes, rinsed and cut into halves
1-2 Tablespoons olive oil
1 teaspoon dried oregano
1 teaspoon minced garlic
1 Tablespoon balsamic vinegar

Preheat oven to 350 degrees F. Mix all ingredients and pour onto a foil-lined baking sheet. Bake 30-45 minutes or until slightly browned and roasted. Serves 1.
Per Serving:
Calories: 194
Carbs: (carbs are from free foods)
Protein: 3gm pro
Fat: 14gm

ROASTED GREEN BEANS WITH ONIONS
12 oz. green beans, fresh, rinsed and stems removed
½ medium onion, thinly sliced
1-2 Tablespoon olive oil
1 Tablespoon balsamic vinegar
½ teaspoon dried thyme leaves (optional)

Preheat oven to 400 degrees. Line a large baking sheet with foil and coat with nonstick spray. Set aside.
In a large bowl, combine all ingredients, mixing well. Sprinkle with salt and pepper as desired.
Spread evenly onto baking sheet. Roast in oven 20-30 minutes until desired tenderness, stirring halfway through roasting time. Serves 4.
Per serving:
Calories: 66
Carbs: (carbs are from free foods)
Protein: 2gm
Fat: 4gm

ROASTED VEGGIES
1 Bunch Asparagus, or other non-starchy vegetables (2 cups), cleaned and trimmed
1-2 Tablespoons Olive Oil
1 teaspoon minced garlic
Salt and pepper, as desired

Preheat oven to 400 degrees F. Line a baking sheet with foil. Combine all ingredients on baking sheet and toss to mix well. Spread asparagus out on pan and roast 10-20 minutes (depending on size of asparagus) or until tender.
Note: Other veggies to roast include squash, peppers, broccoli, cauliflower, etc. If roasting sweet potatoes, peel and cut into chunks or slices, coat lightly with olive oil and roast 20-30 minutes or until tender. Serves 2.
Per Serving:
Calories: 106
Carbs: carbs are from free foods if using non-starchy vegetables- if using sweet potatoes- 15gm carb/ ½ cup serving
Protein: 2gm
Fat: 10gm

DESSERTS

BAKED APPLES

2 small apples
½ cup quick-cooking oats, uncooked
2 Tbsp. butter
1 Tbsp. raisins
1 tsp. cinnamon

Preheat oven to 425°F. Wash apples and remove the cores. In a small bowl, combine the oats, butter, raisins and cinnamon. Stuff the oat mixture into the apples and place in a baking pan. Bake at 425°F for 20 minutes or until tender. Serves 2.
Per Serving:
Calories: 201
Carbs: 29gm
Protein: 4
Fat: 9gm

BAKED PEARS

1 medium Bosc pear
1 teaspoon butter or margarine
1/8 teaspoon cinnamon

Preheat oven to 350 degrees F. Slice pear in half and scoop out seeds. Lay halves cut side up on a baking sheet. (Cut a very small slice under each half to help them sit upright.) Spread butter over halves and sprinkle with cinnamon. Bake for 30-45 minutes or until tender. Serves 2.
Per Serving:
Calories: 72
Carbs: 15gm
Protein: 0
Fat: 1gm

BANANA ICE CREAM

1 large banana

Cut banana into small pieces and place in a freezer bag. Freeze at least 2 hours. Add banana pieces to a small food processor and process until creamy like soft-serve ice cream. Place in a sealed container and freeze until solid. Serves 2.
Per 2.5 oz. Serving:
Calories: 61
Carbs: 16gm
Protein: 1 gm
Fat: 0gm

BERRIES WITH COCONUT AND WHIPPED CREAM

2/3 cup berries
3 Tablespoon unsweetened grated coconut
2 Tablespoons whipped topping

Clean berries and allow to dry. Mix coconut with berries and serve with whipped topping. Serves 1.
Per Serving:
Calories: 168
Carbs: 20gm
Protein: 2gm
Fat: 10gm

BLUEBERRY CRISP

1 cup blueberries, may be frozen
½ Tablespoon whole wheat flour
1 teaspoon honey
¼ cup old fashioned oats- uncooked
½ teaspoon ground cinnamon
½ Tablespoon whole wheat flour
½ Tablespoon honey
1 Tablespoon butter, melted

Preheat oven to 350 degrees. Toss together first 3 ingredients and add to a small baking dish or 3 small ramekins. (Spray dish with non-stick spray.) Mix remaining ingredients and crumble over berries. Bake 20-30 minutes or until oat mixture is golden brown. Allow to cool slightly. Serve with low carb whipped topping if desired. Serves 3.

Per Serving:
Calories: 103
Carbs: 17gm
Protein: 2gm
Fat: 3gm

CHOCOLATE BERRIES

1 Tablespoon semisweet chocolate mini morsels
4 large strawberries
1 Tablespoon chopped walnuts

Melt chocolate and drizzle or spread over berries. Sprinkle with chopped walnuts. Serves 1.
Per Serving:
Calories: 107
Carbs: 15gm
Protein: 1 gm
Fat: 5gm

MISCELLANEOUS

BBQ RUB SEASONING

1 teaspoon sea salt
1 Tablespoon smoked paprika
½ Tablespoon ground black pepper
½ Tablespoon garlic powder
1 teaspoon chili powder

Combine all ingredients and store in an airtight container. Serving = 1 teaspoon
Per Serving:
Calories: 3
Carbs: 0
Protein: 0
Fat: 0

BERRY CRUSH

2 cups mixed berries, frozen
1/3-1/2 cup water

Place berries and water in sauce pan. Bring to a boil and stir/mash berries as syrup forms. Add extra water as needed. May add artificial sweetener to taste as desired. Serves 6.
Per Serving: 2.2 oz.
Calories: 32
Carbs: 8gm
Protein: 1gm
Fat: 0

EASY MARINARA SAUCE

2 (14.5 oz.) cans diced tomatoes with basil, garlic and oregano
1 Tablespoon tomato paste with Italian herbs
1 teaspoon olive oil
1/8 teaspoon ground cinnamon

Place all ingredients in bowl of food processor and pulse until combined and slightly chunky- about 10 seconds. Makes about 3 cups.
Per 8 oz. Serving:
Calories: 52
Carbs: 10gm
Protein: 2gm
Fat: 2gm

PARMESAN CRISPS

½ cup grated parmesan cheese

Preheat oven to 350 degrees F. Line a baking pan with parchment paper. Divide parmesan into 4 rounds and spread cheese out to form a circle. Bake about 7-9 minutes or until melted and golden brown. Loosen from pan and allow to cool.
Per Serving:
Calories: 166
Carbs: 1gm
Protein: 15gm
Fat: 11gm

SMALL BATCH CORNBREAD

1 teaspoon + 1 Tablespoon oil
1/4 cup whole grain cornmeal
1/4 cup unbleached whole grain all-purpose flour
1/4 teaspoon sea salt
1/2 teaspoon baking powder
1/4 teaspoon baking soda
1/3 cup buttermilk
1 egg white

Preheat oven to 425 degrees F. Add 1 teaspoon oil to a 6 1/2" skillet. Place the skillet in the oven as it preheats. In a small bowl, combine cornmeal, flour, salt, baking powder and soda. Stir with a whisk to combine well. Combine buttermilk, egg white and remaining 1 Tablespoon oil. Stir with a whisk to combine well. Pour buttermilk mixture into dry ingredients and stir to combine. When your oven signals it has reached 425 degrees, take the skillet out and pour in the cornbread batter which will sizzle as it spreads in skillet. Return skillet to oven and cook for 15-20 minutes or until top is browned and crispy. Cut into 4 pieces. Serves 4.

Per Serving:

Calories: 103
Carbs: 13 gm
Protein: 3gm
Fat: 4gm

RECIPE INDEX

APPLE NUT SANDWICH	53
BAKED APPLES	83
BAKED PEARS	83
BALSAMIC MUSHROOMS	80
BALSAMIC PORK TENDERLOIN	65
BANANA ICE CREAM	84
BBQ RUB SEASONING	86
BERRIES WITH COCONUT AND WHIPPED CREAM	84
BERRY CRUSH	86
BLUEBERRY CRISP	84
BREAKFAST BANANA SPLIT	56
BREAKFAST BURRITO	56
BROCCOLI TOSS	80
CAESAR SALAD	49
CARIBBEAN COLESLAW	49
CHEESE TOAST	53
CHEESY EGGS	57
CHICKEN (OR PORK) & VEGGIE STIR FRY	65
CHOCOLATE BERRIES	85
CINNAMON TOAST	57
COBB SALAD PLATTER	50
COLESLAW	50
COUNTRY EGG SANDWICH	57
CRUNCHY FISH TACOS CARIBBEAN SLAW	66

DEVILED EGGS	58
EASY BAKED FISH	66
EASY EGGS	58
EASY GREEK CHICKEN	67
EASY GREEK CHICKEN SALAD BOWL	50
EASY MARINARA SAUCE	86
EGG BAKED IN AVOCADO CUPS	59
EGGS BENEDICT	59
EGGS IN HAM CUPS	59
EGGPLANT PARM	67
ENGLISH MUFFIN STACK	60
FAVORITE TACOS	68
FLATBREAD PIZZA	68
FRENCH TOAST	60
FRIED RICE	69
GREEK CHICKEN CHOPPED SALAD	51
GREEK CHICKEN SALAD STUFFED PITA	53
GREEK CHICKEN SANDWICH	54
GREEK CHICKEN WRAP	54
GREEK CHICKEN SALAD	69
GREEK YOGURT PARFAIT	61
GRILLED BBQ PORK CHOP	69
GRILLED SHRIMP WRAP	55
HAM, EGG AND VEGGIE ROLL UP	61
HERB ROASTED CHICKEN & VEGGIES	70
HIGH PROTEIN OATMEAL	62

HUMMUS LUNCH BOWL	70
JERK CHICKEN	71
LIGHTER LASAGNA CAPRESE	71
OAT BOWL	62
OATMEAL BANANA SMOOTHIE	62
OPEN FACED LOADED BURGERS	72
OVEN BAKED BBQ RIBS	72
PARMESAN CRISPS	87
PATTY MELT WITH CARAMELIZED ONIONS	72
PINEAPPLE GRILLED CHICKEN	73
PORK & SPANISH RICE	73
PORK TENDERLOIN WITH APPLES	74
POTATO SKINS	80
RAW VEGGIE PLATE	81
RED & WHITE CHICKEN CHILI	75
ROASTED CHERRY TOMATOES	81
ROASTED GREEN BEANS WITH ONIONS	82
ROASTED VEGGIES	82
ROTISSERIE CHICKEN	75
SALMON PATTIES	76
SMALL BATCH CORNBREAD	87
SPINACH SALAD	51
STEAK KABOBS	76
SUMMER CORN SALAD	52
SWEET POTATO BREAKFAST CUPS	63
TACO SALAD	52

TORTILLA PIZZA	77
TURKEY DIVAN	77
TURKEY MEATSAUCE	78
TURKEY SWISS WRAP	55
VEGGIE OMELET	63
VERACRUZ STYLE SNAPPER	78

Thank you for purchasing this book. Please be sure to check out some of our other titles:

- Easy Diabetes Diet Menus & Grocery Shopping Guide- Menu Me!
- Easy Diabetes Diet Menus- Featuring Mediterranean Favorites ebook
- Diabetes Diet Menus for College Students eBook